The Role of CT Scans in Fighting Esophageal Cancer

Mathew

Contents

Chapter 1.

Introduction

1.1 Contextualization

Esophageal Cancer (EC) is, globally, one of the most frequently reported malignancies [23, 68]. This disease ranks seventh in terms of incidence (572,000 new cases) and sixth in general mortality (509,000 deaths), the latter meaning that EC will account for an estimated one in every 20 deaths from cancer in 2018 [21].

As with other diseases of the upper Gastrointestinal (GI) tract, EC can be evaluated by a variety of imaging modalities [27, 17], including (Figure 1.1):

- Computed Tomography (CT)

    - Application: useful in distinguishing between patients with early cancer who need further evaluation with Endoscopy and those were the tumour is already invading other structures; used for tumour delineation during radiotherapy planning.

    - Main advantages: reliable in determining resectability.

    - Main disadvantages: CT is unable to distinguish the wall layers of the oesophagus to determine the depth of tumour infiltration.

- Positron Emission Tomography (PET)

    - Application: Fluorodeoxyglucose (FDG)-PET is a established imaging technique for staging EC, being the most important role of this modality the detection of distant metastases.

– Main advantages: assessing of metabolic function, high sensibility, high reproducibility (when complying with the acquisition standards), and existence of quantitative measurements such as Standardized Uptake Value (SUV).

– Main disadvantages: low spatial resolution when compared with other techniques, low specificity of 18F-FDG-PET, and a lack of availability of other pharmaceuticals beyond F-18-FDG.

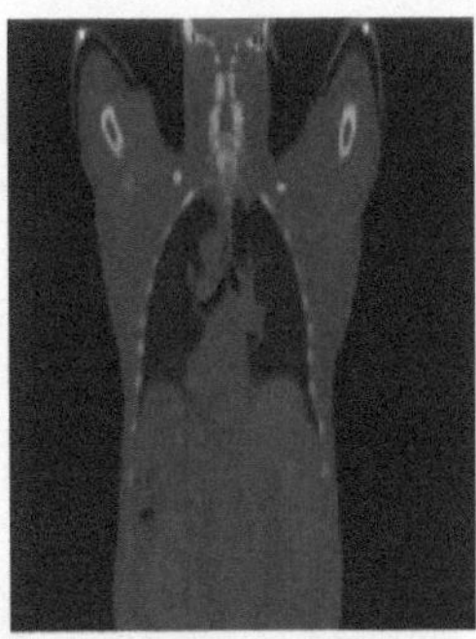

(a) Abdominal CT

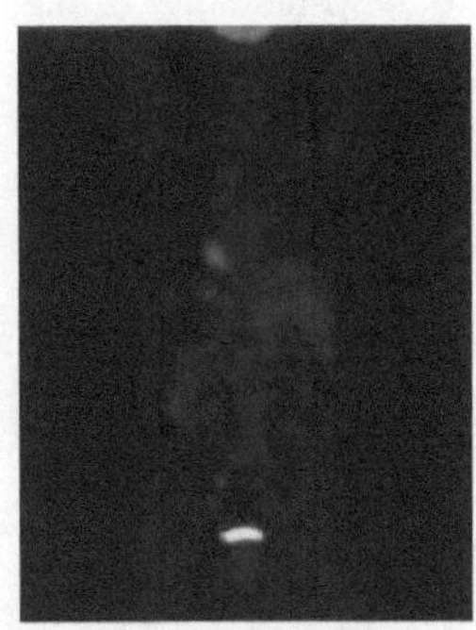

(b) PET imaging

Figure 1.1: EC staging using CT and PET

A summary of the different imaging techniques in EC used in clinical practice for diagnosis, Tumor-Node-Metastasis (TNM)-staging, tumour delineation for Radiotherapy (RT), and treatment response assessment, is given in Table 1.1.

Table 1.1: Imaging techniques in EC used for diagnosis, TNM-staging, tumour delineation for RT, and treatment response assessment [17]

	CT	PET
Diagnosis		
T-Staging	✓	
N-Staging	✓	✓
M-Staging	✓	✓
Tumour delineation for RT	✓	✓
Evaluation of response	✓	✓

Current guidelines for esophageal treatment typically include neoadjuvant radiochemotherapy followed by surgery. In some cases, however, it is known from postsurgery anatomopathologic data, that surgery could be avoided. Computer vision could present solutions aiming at finding criteria for the clear separation between surgical and non-surgical candidates, avoiding the loss of quality of life and surgery associated comorbilities.

The development of these techniques on the present application encompasses two main difficulties. One is the multi-modality of the data. We want to leverage all of the different types of images available, such as PET and CT. The other main difficulty is the existence of small training data. Data augmentation and transfer learning present some possible solutions to this problem.

The present document shows experiments on the classification of PET and CT scans of patients with esophageal cancer into two classes, patients that need surgery and patients that do not need surgery.

1.2 Objectives

This work was presented in the RECPAD 2019 conference and it was submitted to the BIBE 2020 virtual conference (the poster and paper for RECPAD and the BIBE paper can be consulted on appendices B and C). It was developed in the context of the project NORTE-01-0145-FEDER-000027, supported by Norte Portugal Regional Operational Programme (NORTE 2020), under the PORTUGAL 2020 Partnership Agreement, through the European Regional Development Fund (ERDF), whose aim is:

> To develop a comprehensive predictive model of complete response after chemoradiotherapy for patients with EC

The present **book** contributes to that overall aim by:

- Presentation of a new database of patients with oesophagic early-stage cancer, with CT and three PET scans (acquired at different treatment phases) for each patient

- A formalisation of the problem as identification of patients that do not need surgery

- Radiomic and automatic features extracted from both PET and CT

- Traditional learning including fusion at both feature and decision level, feature selection, and several state of the art classifiers

- Different uses of deep learning, as feature extractor, using pre-trained classification networks, and an architecture that was trained from scratch

- Formal evaluation and comparison (both among the best tested methods and with the state of the art works) with their difference measured by a paired sample t-test

1.3 Document Structure

In chapter 2 the foundational knowledge of this book is explained.

Chapter 3 presents not only an overview of the state of the art research on multi-modal approaches to EC data classification but also to the various machine learning models used in such context.

In Chapter 4 there is a description of the dataset that is going to be used for this work, as well as the pipeline for the classification methods implemented in this book. It also describes the various steps the data will go through in order to be usable for the construction of the various machine learning algorithms.

In Chapter 5 the "traditional" machine learning classification algorithms will be constructed and tested on the data and their results discussed.

Then, in Chapter 6 a deep learning model will be constructed with the data and its results will also be discussed.

In Chapter 7 the results from "traditional" and deep learning algorithms will be compared.

The document finishes in Chapter 8 with some conclusions and possible suggestions for future work.

Chapter 2.

Background Knowledge

2.1 Esophageal cancer

Esophageal cancer remains one of the deadliest cancers worldwide (509,000 deaths), with an overall 5-year survival rate of less than 18%. It is also one of the most incident cancers, with an estimated 17,990 new cases in the United States in 2013 [71]. The incidence and mortality rates in men is 2 to 3 times larger than in women, as approximately 70% occur in the former, with the mortality rates among men in developed countries also being 2 times greater. This type of cancer is more common in Eastern and Southern African countries, being the leading cause of cancer mortality in Kenyan men [21]. Genetic and dietary factors are also at fault: smoking and alcohol have been strongly associated with Squamous Cell Carcinoma (SCC) and gastroesophageal reflux disease has been associated with Barrett esophagus and adenocarcinoma [52].

2.1.1 Anatomy

The esophagus is approximately 20 to 30 cm in length and it extends from the hypopharynx to the stomach, posterior to the trachea and the heart, passing through the esophageal hiatus, and is composed of three general layers: the mucosa, the submucosa and muscularis propria. It is also divided into three anatomical areas (Figure 2.1), comprising cervical, upper and middle thoracic, and lower thoracic/esophagogastric junction [71]:

1. The cervical esophagus extends from the esophageal orifice to the sternal notch. Endoscopic measurements range from 15 to 20 cm.

2. The upper thoracic esophagus extends from the sternal notch to the azygos vein arch. Typically, it is located from 20 to 25 cm from the incisors. Endoscopic measurements range from 25 to 30 cm.

3. The lower thoracic esophagus extends from below the inferior pulmonary vein to the gastroesophageal junction (Gastroesophageal Junction (GEJ)). Endoscopic measurements range from 30 to 40 cm.

The esophagus also has a pattern of rich and dense interconnected network of lymphatic vessels deep within submucosa that communicate with the lymphatics of the muscular layers. Lymphatic channels in the submucosa facilitate the spread of neoplastic cells along the esophageal wall [71].

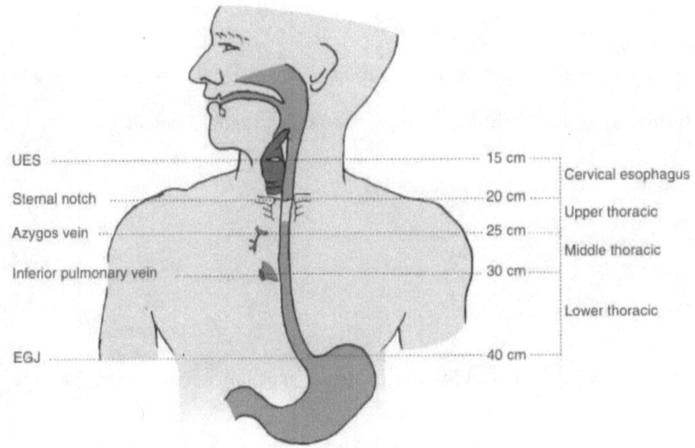

Figure 2.1: Anatomic landmarks of the esophagus: GEJ and Upper Esophageal Sphincter (UES) [71]

2.1.2 Histologic types

Esophageal cancer is classified in two subtypes: Adenocarcinoma (AC) and SCC. Adenocarcinomas tend to involve the distal third of the esophagus and the gastroesophageal junction, whereas SCCs are usually located in the upper and middle thirds of the esophagus [71]. Adenocarcinoma is a malignant epithelial tumor with glandular differentiation arising from Barrett esophagus mucosa in the lower third of the esophagus. They might also originate from heterotropic gastric mucosa in the upper esophagus or from mucosal and submucosal glands.

Squamous cell carcinoma is also a malignant epithelial tumour but with squamous cell differentiation, characterized by keratinocyte-like cells with intercellular bridges and/or keratinization [71]. These two subtypes are assumed to have different biological behaviors, so it is important to determine the tumor location and confirm the histological cell type.

2.1.3 Tumor, Node and Metastasis staging

The TNM staging system was created by Pierre Denoix circa 1943 and 1952 and is currently maintained and developed by the American Joint Committee on Cancer (AJCC) and the Union for International Cancer Control (UICC). It classifies and groups cancers by the extent of local tumor invasion into the esophageal wall and advanced invasion into adjacent structures (T), the status of regional draining lymph nodes (N) and the presence or absence of distant metastases (M).

In the T-stage the depth of the invasion into the four distinct layers (involving the esophageal wall and adventitia) is assessed, according to the following nomenclature:

- TX: Primary tumor cannot be assessed

- T0: No evidence of primary tumor

- Tis: High-grade dysplasia

- T1: Tumor invading mucosal lamina propria, muscularis mucosae or submucosa

    - T1a: Tumor invading into the lamina propria or muscularis mucosae

    - T1b: Tumor invading submucosa

- T2: Tumor invading muscularis propria

- T3: Tumor invading adventitia

- T4: Tumor invading adjacent structures

    - T4a: Resectable tumor invading pleura, pericardium or diaphragm

    - T4b: Unresectable tumor invading other adjacent structures, such as aorta, vertebral body or trachea

This staging is crucial to determining suitability for surgical resection (i.e., if the tumor can be surgically removed or not).

The nodal classification (N) is the most controversial of the stages, since there is no consensus on the ideal number of nodes that must be resected for optimal surgery. The presence of lymph node metastases is a major prognostic indicator, as patients without lymph node metastases have an overall 5-year survival rate of 70-92% when treated by surgical resection, but this falls to 18-47% if metastases are pathologically confirmed. It is defined as follows:

- N0: No positive node

- N1: 1 to 2 nodes

- N2: 3 to 6 nodes

- N3: 7 or more nodes

The likelihood of distant metastases increases with advanced T and N-stages. If distant metastases disease is detected on cross-sectional imaging, the patient receives palliative therapy unless specific oligo-metastatic can be resected. This stage (M) is simply designated as:

- M0: no distant metastasis

- M1: distant metastasis

2.2 Medical Image Modalities

Multimodal imaging in biomedicine is a well estabilished diagnosis method in cancer patients, as different image modalities offer new information about the tumor-induced tissue that can be complementary to each other. In esophageal cancer diagnosis [71], the standard modalities include Upper Endoscopy, Computer Tomography (CT) scans, Positron Emission Tomography (PET) scans, Endoscopic Ultrasound (EUS) and, in selected patients, Magnetic Resonance Imaging (MRI), endoscopic mucosal resections, endobronchial ultrasounds and thoracoscopic/laparoscopic procedures. However, the focus of this book will be on CT and PET.

2.2.1 Computed Tomography

Although it is often complemented with Endoscopic Ultrasound (EUS) regarding the assessment of T stage [67], Computed Tomography scan (CT) is typically the first radiological test applied after the esophageal cancer diagnosis via Endoscopy. It displays the lesion, surrounding structures, lymph node metastasis and regional organ invasion and it has an important role in detecting distant metastasis [71]. In Figures 2.2 and 2.3 are shown examples of an adenocarcinoma and SCC detected by CT scan.

However, its main limitation lies in its insensitivity in identifying metastatic disease in normal-sized lymph nodes; it also cannot distinguish between T1, T2 and T3 stages [67], even though it is useful for excluding unresectable tumor (T4) disease, as it is detected in up to 30% of patients [71].

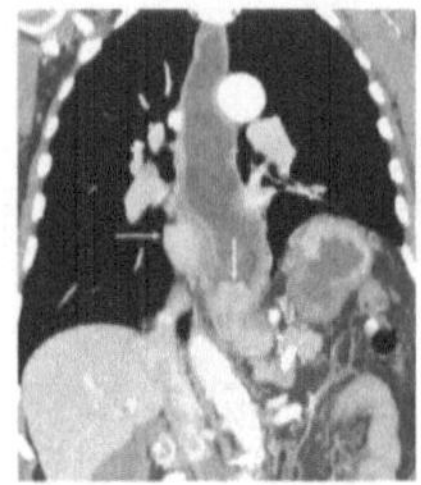

Figure 2.2: CT image of an adenocarcinoma of the GEJ. The white arrow shows a partially obstructing mass at the gastroesophageal junction, while the yellow arrow points to a paraesophageal adenopathy [71]

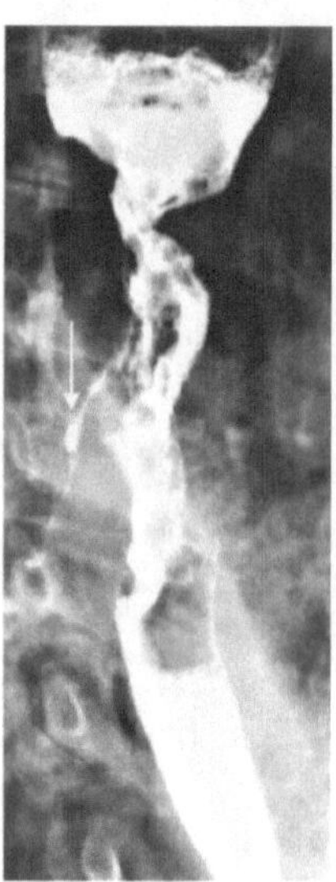

Figure 2.3: Squamous cell carcinoma of the midesophagus. The white arrow points to a possible esophageal-bronchial fistula [71]

2.2.2 Positron Emission Tomography

This type of image modality has gained popularity as a noninvasive method for the staging of esophageal cancer, particularly for the detection of distant metastasis, with a sensitivity ranging from 70% to 74% [67].

PET scans work by highlighting the metabolically active tissue via a glucose analogue (2-fluoro-2-deoxyglucose, or FDG), which remains trapped in cancer cells during metabolism, due to FDG-6-phosphate (in contrast to glucose-6-phosphate) not being a substrate for further metabolism in the glycolytic pathway, and it enters the cells via the same membrane transporters as glucose. Both glucose and FDG arethen phosphorylated by the enzyme hexokinase [71].

Due to the insufficient esophageal wall definition provided by this type of image modality (Figures 2.4 and 2.5), PET has no value in T staging. It also has poor spatial resolution, which in turns renders it insufficient to separate the primary tumor from juxtatumoral lymph nodes. Its ability in identifying lymph node involvement is also lackluster, with a sensitivity ranging from 38% to 82%. According to a study mentioned in [71], the sensitivities for node detection are as follows (respectively):

- Cervical, upper thoracic and abdominal nodes: 78%, 82% and 60%;

- Mid and lower mediastinum: 38% and 0%.

whereas the specificity of this image modality is considerably better than its sensitivity for N staging, ranging from 76% to 95%, compared to CT's 77% to 89% [71].

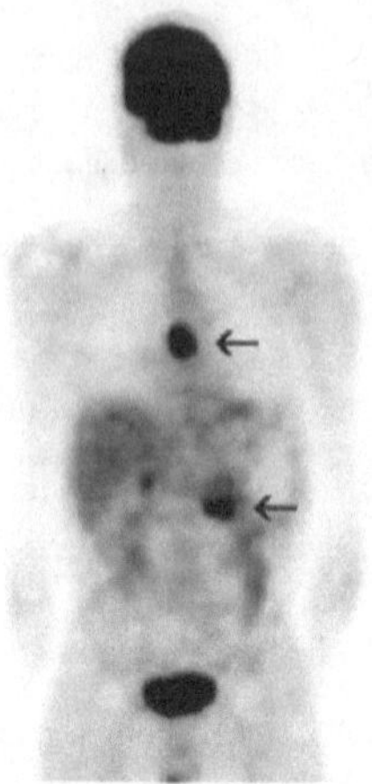

Figure 2.4: FDG-PET scan on a patient with a synchronous carcinoma in the mid esophagus (first arrow) and a Grawitz's carcinoma on the left kidney [67]

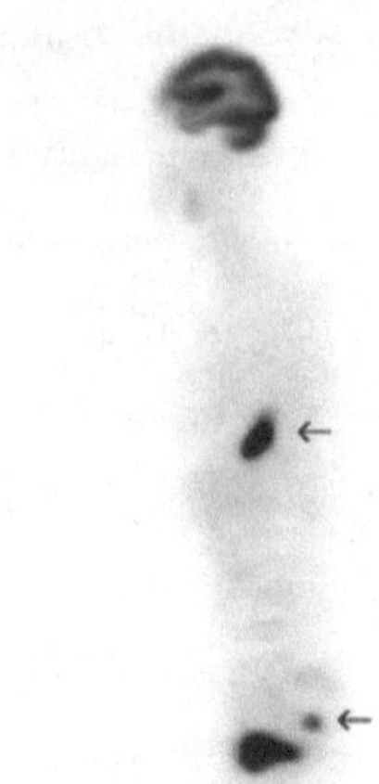

Figure 2.5: FDG-PET scan on a patient with a distal esophageal tumor and a synchronous rectal adenoma [67]

PET's main utility lies in identifying distant metastasis' presence, as compared with CT alone. Luketich *et al.* [37] reported the percentages of sensitivity, specificity and accuracy for CT and PET, as described in Table 2.1.

Table 2.1: Luketich *et al.* [37] study of sensitivity, specificity and accuracy of PET and CT

	CT	PET
Sensitivity (%)	46.1	69.0
Specificity (%)	73.8	93.4
Accuracy (%)	63.0	84.0

2.3 Machine Learning

In the field of biomedical imaging, statistical learning methods are often used for feature extraction and classification. In this section, the "traditional" and deep learning methods used in the context of this **book** will be further explained, as well as evaluation methodologies for the constructed models.

2.3.1 Traditional Learning

k-Nearest Neighborhoods

Nearest-neighbor classifiers are based on **learning by analogy**, i.e., comparing a given feature vector with others in the training set that are similar to it [34]. Each feature vector is described by n attributes, i.e.:

$$x_i = (x_1, ..., x_n) \tag{2.1}$$

and each vector represents a point in an n-dimensional space. Thus, all of the feature vectors are stored in an n-dimensional pattern space. Given a feature vector **X**, a **k-nearest neighbor** classifier searches the k nearest training examples closest to it and returns the majority label(i.e., the predominant label of the training examples **X** is closest to) [8].

The "closeness" of two vectors is defined in terms of a distance metric, such as the Euclidean distance [34], which is defined by Equation 2.2 :

$$dist(X1, X2) = \sqrt{\sum_{i=1}^{n}(x_{1i} - x_{2i})^2} \tag{2.2}$$

where X_1 and X_2 are feature vectors, $x_{1i_{i=1}^{n}}$ and $x_{2i_{i=1}^{n}}$ their respective attributes.

Naive Bayes

The Naive Bayes method is a probabilistic classifier, i.e., it quantifies the relationship between a case and the class it belongs to as a probability. It is based on the Bayes Theorem for conditional probabilities [34]:

$$P(A|B) = \frac{P(B|A) \cdot P(A)}{P(B)} \tag{2.3}$$

where:

- $P(A)$ and $P(B)$ are the probabilities of events A and B, respectively;

- $P(A|B)$ is the probability of A given B;

- $P(B|A)$ is the probability of B given A.

Naive Bayesian Classifiers work on the class-conditional independence assumption, i.e., it assumes that the effect of an attribute value on a given class is independent of the values of the other attributes, given by [34]:

$$P(x_1, ..., x_n|y_j) = \prod_{k=1}^{n} P(x_k|y_j)$$

This assumption is made to simplify the calculations involved, thus considered "naïve" in this sense. However, it is highly accurate and fast when applied to large databases [34].

Discriminant Analysis

Fisher's Linear Discriminant Analysis (1936) is a binary classification method that works as follows: given a dataset with two classes, it will determine the best set of features of both of them in order to separate between the two. This method operates on finding a function that discriminates between the two classes but, instead of a hyperplane, it uses a linear one-dimensional function of the form [5]

$$f(x) = w^T x + b \tag{2.4}$$

to separate the two classes, which in turn is called a **linear discriminant function**. It can be said that a given input x belongs to class 1 if $f(x) > 0$ and to class 2 if $f(x) \leq 0$ [5].

Let μ_1, μ_2 be the centers of classes 1 and 2 (respectively) and $\hat{\mu}_1, \hat{\mu}_2$ their projections on a one-dimensional linear subspace (also respectively). The deviation of the projected points will be [5]:

$$(\hat{\mu}_1 - \hat{\mu}_2)^2 = (\frac{w^T \mu_1}{||w||} - \frac{w^T \mu_2}{||w||})^2 = (\frac{w^T}{||w||}(\mu_1 - \mu_2))^2 \tag{2.5}$$

which will be maximixed when w has the same direction of $\mu_1 - \mu_2$. LDA's main idea is to consider the entire data's covariance matrix projection onto a one-dimensional linear subspace which maximizes the variance of the projected centers, while simultaneously minimizes the variance of the projected data points within each class. The optimization problem is then the *max ratio problem*, given by [5]:

$$\max_{w} \frac{(\hat{\mu}_1 - \hat{\mu}_2)^2}{s_1^2 + s_2^2} \tag{2.6}$$

where

$$s_1^2 = \frac{1}{l_1 - 1} \sum_{x_i \in C_1} (\hat{x}_i - \hat{\mu}_1) \tag{2.7}$$

and

$$s_2^2 = \frac{1}{l_2 - 1} \sum_{x_i \in C_2} (\hat{x}_i - \hat{\mu}_2) \tag{2.8}$$

represent the scaled variance of the projected points within each class (respectively) and $\hat{x} := f(x) := \frac{w^T}{||w||}x + b$ is the projection. One can also assume the constraints $||w|| = 1$ and $s_1^2 + s_2^2 = 1$; the problem is then solved using Lagrange's multiplier's [5].

Decision Trees

Decision trees are a classification method where the classification process is performed using a set of hierarchial decisions of the feature variables, arranged in a tree-like structure. In each node, a *split criterion* is applied in order to divide the data into two of more parts [34]. There are several types of decision-tree algorithms, such as Iterative Dichotomizer 3 (ID3), C4.5 and Classification and Regression Trees (CART) [34]. For this **book**, the latter will be used.

The goal of this method is to identify a split criterion in order to minimize the level of "mixing" of the class variables. Each node in the decision tree is a partition of the data space defined by the combination of the split criteria in the nodes above it. A decision tree has two types of nodes [34]:

- **Internal node:** contains a test over the value of a prediction variable;

- **Leaf node:** contains the value of the class.

The standard split criterion used for the CART algorithm is the **Gini Index** [1]. The Gini Index of a dataset D where each data point belongs to one of the c classes is given by:

$$Gini(D) = 1 - \sum_{i=1}^{c} p_i^2$$

where p_i is the probability of class i.

The overall Gini index for an r-way split of a set S into its r subsets may be quantified as the weighted average of the Gini index of each S_i, where the weight of S_i is $|S_i|$:

$$Gini - Split(S \implies S_1, ..., S_r) = \sum_{i=1}^{r} \frac{|S_i|}{|S|} Gini(S_i)$$

The split with the lowest Gini index of its alternatives is then selected. Moreover, if a tree grows too large in size, it may lead to **overfitting**, i.e., the algorithm will not generalize well to unseen data [1].

Pruning is then applied to the tree in order to remove branches that may be hindering the tree's efficiency. Normally, it is not possible to have *a priori* knowledge of when to prune the tree, therefore the most common practice is letting the tree grow overly large and then prune unreliable branches according to a pre-defined statistical procedure (also known as *post-pruning*) [34].

Support Vector Machines

Support Vector Machine (SVM) is a binary classification method for both linear and non-linear data, and it operates by using a nonlinear mapping to transform the data into a higher dimension. Within this new dimension, it utilizes a decision boundary known as the **separating hyperplane** to separate the data into two classes. SVMs find this hyperplane by using support vectors and margins (defined by the former), concepts which will be explained later on [34].

Let $D = \{(X_i, y_i)\}_{i=1}^{|D|}$ be a dataset, where X_i is a feature vector associated with class label $y_i \in -1, +1$. D is **linearly separable** if there is a hyperplane (in this case, a straight line) that separates all feature vectors by their respective classes, which is given by [34]:

$$w \cdot x - b = 0 \qquad (2.9)$$

where:

- **w** is a weight vector;

- **x** is a feature vector;

- **b** is a bias.

However, there are infinite possibilities of constructing a separating hyperplane between the two classes. Therefore, the "best" hyperplane (i.e., the one that minimizes the classification error). SVMs approach this issue by searching for the **Maximum Margin Hyperplane (MMH)**. Using Figure 2.6 as an example, it can be seen that both hyperplanes correctly classify the data; however, it is expected that the one with the largest margin will be the most accurate [34].

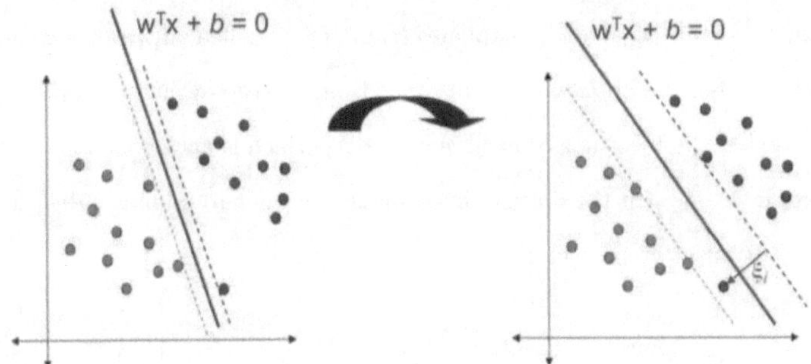

Figure 2.6: Two separating hyperplanes with varying margin sizes. ξ_i represents the error in the training data. [50]

The MMH is determined by rewriting 2.9 (where $n = |D|$) as [34]:

$$\sum_{i=1}^{n} w_i \cdot x_i - b = 0 \qquad (2.10)$$

Thus, any point lying above the separating hyperplane satisfies:

$$\sum_{i=1}^{n} w_i \cdot x_i - b > 0 \tag{2.11}$$

Similarly, any point lying above the separating hyperplane satisfies [34]:

$$\sum_{i=1}^{n} w_i \cdot x_i - b < 0 \tag{2.12}$$

The weights can be adjusted so that the hyperplanes that define the "sides" of the margin can be written as [34]:

$$H_1 = \sum_{i=1}^{n} w_i \cdot x_i - b \geq 1, y_i = +1 \tag{2.13}$$

and

$$H_2 = \sum_{i=1}^{n} w_i \cdot x_i - b \leq 1, y_i = -1 \tag{2.14}$$

Both equations can, however, be combined to form [34]:

$$y_i \cdot \left(\sum_{i=1}^{n} w_i \cdot x_i - b \right) \geq 1 \tag{2.15}$$

Any feature vectors that fall on hyperplanes H_1 or H_2 are called **support vectors**. A formula for the MMH can now be obtained: the distance from the separating hyperplane to any point on H_1 is $\frac{1}{||w||}$, where $||w||$ is the Euclidean norm of W, which is analogous for H_2; therefore, the maximal margin is $\frac{2}{||w||}$. For the optimal hyperplane, we want to minimize $||w||$, which leads to the following optimization problem [34]:

$$\text{minimize } ||w||, \text{ s.t. } y_i \left(\sum_{i=1}^{n} w_i \cdot x_i - b \right) \geq 1, (i = 1, ..., n) \tag{2.16}$$

The linear SVM approach can be extended to create nonlinear SVMs for nonlinear data classification. This new linear approach consists of two main steps [34]:

1. Transform the data into a higher dimension using a nonlinear mapping by using the Kernel

Trick: when solving the linear SVM optimization problem 2.16, the feature vectors appear in the form of dot products, $\phi(x_i) \cdot \phi(x_j)$, where $\phi(x)$ is the nonlinear function applied to transform the feature vectors. As dot product computation is extremely heavy on high-dimensional spaces, applying a **Kernel function**, $K(x_i, x_j)$, to the original data is not only mathematically equivalent to the dot product but also considerably more efficient. That is:

$$K(x_i, x_j) = \phi(x_i) \cdot \phi(x_j) \tag{2.17}$$

Examples of Kernel functions include:

- **Polynomial kernel:** $k(x_i, x_j) = (x_i \cdot x_j + 1)^d$

- **Gaussian kernel:** $k(x_i, x_j) = \exp \frac{||x_i - x_j||}{2 \cdot \sigma^2}$

- **Sigmoid kernel:** $k(x_i, x_j) = tanh(\kappa x_i \cdot x_j + \delta)$

2. After applying this trick, a search for the optimal hyperplane is performed. The procedure is similar to 2.16, although it involvess placing a regularization term C, which controls the trade-off between maximizing the margin and minimizing the *noise* (or error) in the training data, ξ_i. Thus, 2.16 can now be rewritten as [66]:

$$\text{minimize } ||w|| + C \cdot \sum_{i=1}^{n} \xi_i, \text{ s.t. } y_i(\sum_{i=1}^{n} w_i \cdot x_i - b) \geq 1 - \xi_i, (i = 1, ..., n) \tag{2.18}$$

Ensemble Models

Ensemble models are an approach to increase the prediction accuracy by combining the results from multiple classifiers. This classification method is motivated by the fact that different classifiers may make different predictions due to their specific characteristics or their sensitivity to small variations in the data. The results are then combined into a single robust prediction [1].

Bagging (short for *bootstrap aggregating*) is a type of ensemble model that creates various models on different random samples of the original dataset. These samples are taken uniformly with replacement and are known as *bootstrap samples*. Since the random sampling is done with replacement, the bootstrap sample will contain duplicates (in general), therefore some of the original data points will be missing even if the bootstrap sample is of the same size as the original dataset, which will create diversity among the models in the ensemble [26].

This ensemble method is useful in combination with tree models, which are sensitive to variations in the training data. The application of bagging to tree models also encompasses another idea: to build each tree from a different random subset of the features, a process referred to as **subspace sampling**. This in turn encourages the diversity in the ensemble even more, and has the additional advantage that the training time is reduced for each tree. The resulting ensemble method is called *random forest* [26] .

2.3.2 Feature Selection

Feature selection algorithms reduce the dataset's dimension by selecting only a subset of predictor variables to create a model. These algorithms search for a subset of predictors that optimally model measured responses, subject to constraints (e.g., size of subset and required features). With this, prediction performance is improved and faster and more cost-effective predictors are provided. The two types of feature selection algorithms used in this **book** were the **Filter Type** and **Wrapper Type** algorithms, which will now be discussed.

Filter Type feature selection algorithms [42] measure feature importance based on the characteristics of the features (such as variance and response relevance). The following filter type algorithms were used:

- **Neighborhood Component Analysis (NCA):** Let $S = \{(x_i, y_i), i = 1, ..., n\}$ be a training set with n observations, where $x_i \in \mathbb{R}^p$ and $y_i \in \{1, 2, ..., c\}$ (where c is the number of classes). The goal is to learn a classifier $f : \mathbb{R}^p \longrightarrow \{1, 2, ..., c\}$ such that $f(x)$ is the label prediction for the true class of feature vector x [43].

  Let now be considered a randomized classifier that:

  - Randomly picks a reference point for x, $Ref(x)$, from S;

  - Labels x using the label of $Ref(x)$.

  Similar to the K-Nearest Neighborhood (K-NN) algorithm, the reference point is chosen to be the "nearest neighbor" of x, the difference being that, in NCA, it is randomly chosen and all points in S have a probability of being chosen, given by Equation 2.19 [43]:

$$P(Ref(x) = x_j|s) \tag{2.19}$$

where x_j is a point in S. The probability of x_j being picked as the reference point for x is higher if x_j is closer to x as measured by the distance function in Equation 2.20 [43]:

$$d_w(x_i, x_j) = \sum_{r=1}^{p} w_r^2 |x_{ir} - x_{jr}| \tag{2.20}$$

where w_r is the feature's weights. Suppose now that Equation 2.19 can be expressed as a kernel function that takes 2.20 as an argument, and assumes large values when it is small. Equation 2.19 can be written as

$$P(Ref(x) = x_j|S) = \frac{k(d_w(x_i, x_j))}{\sum_{j=1, j\neq i}^{n} k(d_w(x_i, x_j))} \tag{2.21}$$

as the reference point for x is chosen from S, therefore the sum of 2.19, for all j, must be equal to 1 [43]. Applying the leave-one-out method, i.e., predicting y_i using the data in S^{-i} (S without (x_i, y_i)). The probability that point x_j is picked as the reference point is [43]:

$$p_{ij} = P(Ref(x) = x_j|S^{-i}) = \frac{k(d_w(x_i, x_j))}{\sum_{j=1, j\neq i}^{n} k(d_w(x_i, x_j))} \tag{2.22}$$

The probability p_i of correctly classifying i using S^{-i} is given by Equatio n 2.23:

$$p_i = \sum_{j=1, j\neq i}^{n} P(Ref(x) = x_j|S^{-i})I(y_i = y_j) = \sum_{j=1, j\neq i}^{n} p_{ij}y_{ij} \tag{2.23}$$

where

$$y_{ij} = \begin{cases} 1 & y_i = y_j \\ 0 & otherwise \end{cases}$$

- **ReliefF:** this algorithm penalizes the predictor that give different results to neighbors of the same class, rewarding predictors that give different values to neighbors of different classes. Firstly, all predictor weights W_j are set to 0. Then, the algorithm iteratively selects a random observation x_r, finds the k-nearest observation to x_r for each class and updates, for each nearest neighbor x_q, all the weights for the predictors F_j as [44]:

$$W_j^i = W_j^{i-1} - \frac{\Delta_j(x_r, x_q)}{m} \cdot d_{rq} \tag{2.24}$$

for x_r and x_q in the same class, and as:

$$W_j^i = W_j^{i-1} + \frac{P_{yq}}{1 - P_{yr}} \cdot \frac{\Delta_j(x_r, x_q)}{m} \cdot d_{rq} \tag{2.25}$$

where:

- W_j^i is the weight of F_j and the i-th step

- p_{yr} and p_{yq} are the prior probabilities of x_r and x_q's classes (respectively);

- m is the number of iterations

- $\frac{\Delta_j(x_r, x_q)}{m} \cdot d_{rq}$ is the difference of F_j's value between x_r and x_q (x_{rj} and x_{qj} denote the j-th predictor's values in each observation). it is given by Equation 2.26:

$$\frac{\Delta_j(x_r, x_q)}{m} \cdot d_{rq} = \frac{|x_{rj} - x_{qj}|}{max(F_i) - min(F_j)} \tag{2.26}$$

- d_{rq} is a distance function of the form:

$$d_{rq} = \frac{\tilde{d}_{rq}}{\sum_{l=1}^{n} \tilde{d}_{rl}} \tag{2.27}$$

where $\tilde{d}_{rq}$ is a scaling factor, given by:

$$\tilde{d}_{rq} = e^{-(\frac{rank(r,q)}{sigma})^2} \tag{2.28}$$

with $rank(r, q)$ being the position of the q-th observation among the number of nearest neighbors of the r-th observation, and "sigma" being specified by the user [44].

- **Wrapper Type feature selection:** this type of algorithms start by using a subset of features and then add (or remove) a feature using a selection criterion, which measures the change in model performance that results from adding or removing a feature. The algorithm repeats until some stopping criteria are met [45]. **Sequential Feature Selection** was the wrapper type algorithm used in this book, and it has two components [45]:

- **Objective function:** also called the **criterion**, the method seeks to minimize it over all feasible feature subsets;

- **Sequential search algorithm:** adds or removes features from a candidate subset while evaluating the criterion. it is computationally unfeasible to iterate through all possible subset combinations, as a set with n would have 2^n possible subsets. For this, the sequential search algorithm only moves in one direction and it has two variants:

  * **Forward selection:** features are sequentially added to an empty set until the addition of features does not decrease the criterion;

  * **Backward selection:** features are sequentially removed from a full candidate set until the removal of features does not increase the criterion.

2.3.3 Deep Learning

Deep learning algorithms are seeing their rise in use on the artificial intelligence field, most notably in self-driving cars, image recognition and in biomedical image processing and evaluation (i.e., the context of this **book**) to excellent degrees of accuracy. In this section, background knowledge about neural networks and deep learning will be explored.

Neuron

Neural networks are composed of various types of interconnected **neurons**, which work by receiving input from one or more sources ($X = (x_1, ..., x_n)$), which are then multiplied by a set of weights ($W = (w_1, ..., w_n)$) and a bias ($b = (b_1, ..., b_n)$) is added to it. Finally, the previous sum is passed through an activation function [33]. Figure 2.7 shows an example of an artificial neuron.

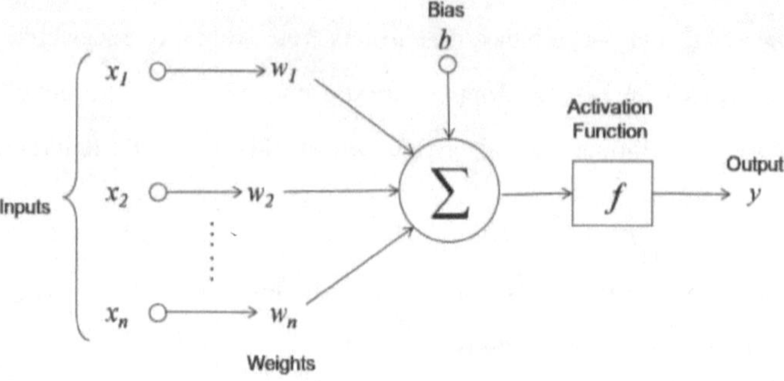

Figure 2.7: An artificial Neuron [46]

As specified earlier, the neurons can have various roles within a neural network. The three main types [33] are:

- **Input neurons:** these neurons are the placeholders for the data given to the neural network;

- **Hidden neurons:** receive input from other neurons (input or other hidden ones) and help the network understand the input and form the output;

- **Output neurons:** provide the processed data from the network

Activation Function

Choosing an activation function is of paramount importance, as it directly affects the performance of the neural network by estabilishing bounds for the neurons' outputs. The most commonly used activation functions will therefore be discussed:

- **Linear Activation Function:** Given by 2.29, this function outputs exactly what the neuron inputs passed to it [33].

$$\phi(x) = x \tag{2.29}$$

It is more commonly used in regression neural networks, i.e., those that learn to provide numeric values. Figure 2.8 shows a graphical representation of this activation function

[33].

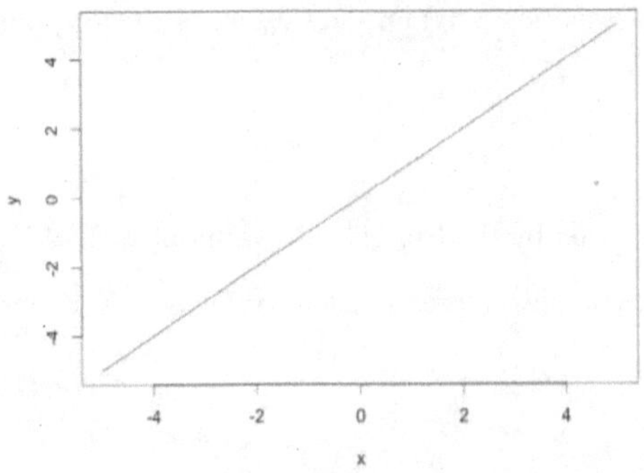

Figure 2.8: Linear activation function graph [33]

- **Step Activation Function:** Given by Equation 2.30, the step (or threshold) activation function returns 1 (true) for values above the specified threshold, and 0 otherwise (0.5 is arbitrary) [33]:

$$\phi(x) = \begin{cases} 1 & x \geq 0.5 \\ 0 & x < 0.5 \end{cases} \tag{2.30}$$

A graphical representation can be seen in Figure 2.9.

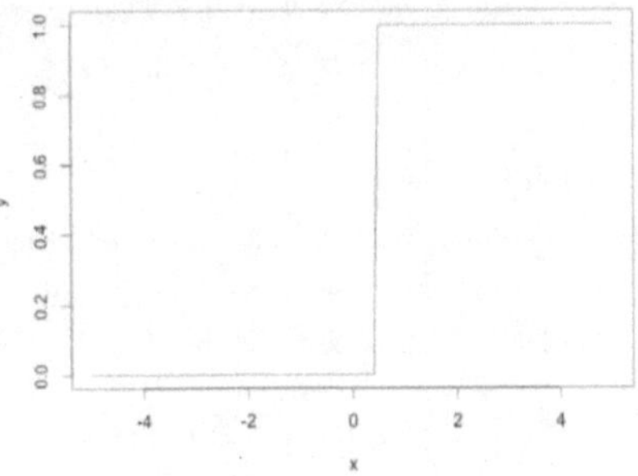

Figure 2.9: Step activation function graph [33]

- **Sigmoid Activation Function:** Widely used in binary classification problems, this function (given by Equation 2.31) outputs values in the [0,1] range [33].

$$\phi(x) = \frac{1}{1 + e^{-x}} \tag{2.31}$$

It is commonly replaced by the **hyperbolic tangent** or **ReLU** functions, which will be explained later. A graphical representation can be seen in Figure 2.10.

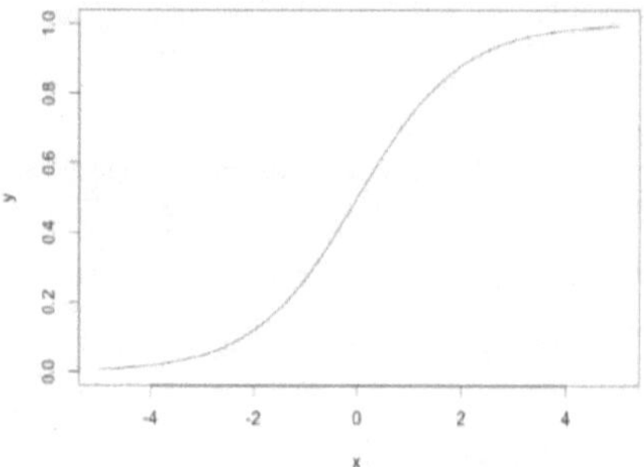

Figure 2.10: Sigmoid activation function graph [33]

- **Hyperbolic Tangent Activation Function:** This function (Equation 2.32) is an alternative to the previous one, and it takes values in the [-1,1] range [33].

$$\phi(x) = \frac{e^x - e^{-x}}{e^x + e^{-x}} \tag{2.32}$$

Its graphical representation is shown in Figure 2.11.

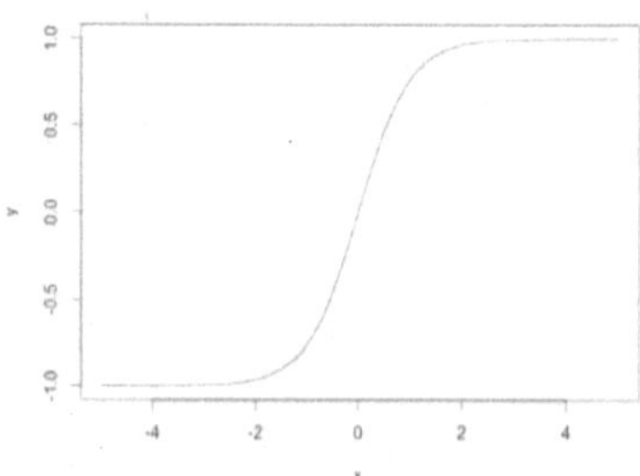

Figure 2.11: Hyperbolic tangent activation function graph [33]

- **Rectified Linear United (ReLU) Activation Function:** Given by Equation 2.33, this function is the most commonly used in neural network implementations, as it performs considerably better than the previously discussed functions [33].

$$\phi(x) = max(0, x) \tag{2.33}$$

The improved performance is, in part, due to the fact that it does not converge to any particular value, unlike its hyperbolic tangent and sigmoid counterparts, which converge to either -1, 0 or 1[33]. A graphical representation is shown in Figure 2.12

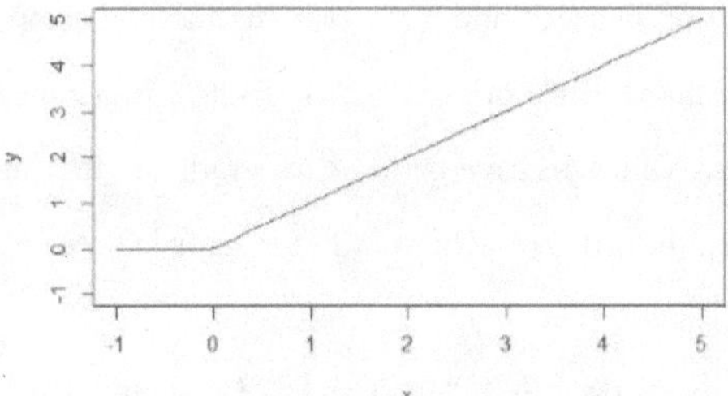

Figure 2.12: ReLU activation function graph [33]

- **Softmax Activation Function:** Given by Equation 2.34, the softmax function is typically used in classification networks and it converts its input to a probability of it belonging to a certain class [33].

$$\phi_i(z) = \frac{e^{z_i}}{\sum_{j \in group} e^{z_j}} \tag{2.34}$$

One neuron per class is needed to classify the data, and the one with the highest value claims the input as a member of its class.

Figure 2.13 shows an example of a neural network. So far, only the neurons and activation functions of a neural network were discussed. Knowledge about backpropagation and gradient descent will now be discussed.

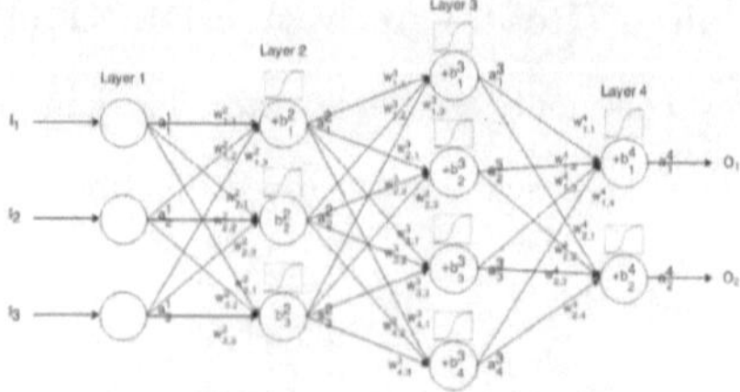

Figure 2.13: Example on an artificial neuron network [49]. Layer 1 is the input layer (i.e., where the input neurons are located), Layers 2 and 3 are the hidden layers and Layer 4 is the output layer. The graphs above each neuron are the activation function of each one of them (in this case, the hyperbolic tangent), the $\omega_{i,j}$'s are the weights and the b_i's are the biases. Biases may or may not be squared.

Gradient Descent and Backpropagation

Gradient descent refers to the calculation of a gradient on each weight in the network for each training example. The gradient is essentially the partial derivative of each weight in the network, and its calculation helps decide if the training method should increase or decrease the weight, therefore decreasing the network's error. A gradient of 0 indicates that the weight is not contributing to the error, while positive or negative gradients indicate that it should decrease (or increase, respectively) in order to achieve a lower error [33]. An illustration can be seen on Figure 2.14.

Essentially, training methods search for the set of weights that minimize the error for a training set. An exhaustive search for all weights is too computationally expensive to be a viable option, so the alternative is to determine the slope of the error function's curve at a certain weight. In conclusion, the gradient is the slope of the error function (which measures the distance of the neural network output to the expected output) and the derivative at that point gives the gradient. Each derivative is calculated using the chain rule of calculus, and each weight is considered an independent variable, as they change independently as the network also changes [33].

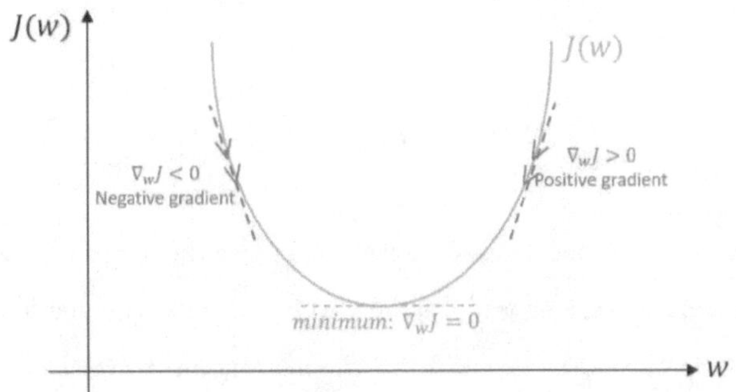

Figure 2.14: Gradient descent example, where $J(w)$ is the cost function [12]

The **backpropagation** algorithm adjusts the neural network's weights with their respective gradients, hereby reducing the global error during training [33].

There are three different ways [33] of approaching this task:

- **Online training:** the weights are modified after each training example. The gradients obtained in the first example are used to change the weights, then the training progresses to the next example and calculates an update to the neural network, iterating through all of the training examples, until all of them are used;

- **Batch training:** the gradients of each training set element are summed and then the network's weights are updated. A batch size is normally set so that training can be more efficient. E.g., for a 1000 element training set, 100-sized batches can be set and the weights will be updated 10 times during training;

- **Stochastic Gradient Descent (SGD):** this algorithm works in either Batch or Online mode. The batch mode works by randomly choosing a batch size; then, the gradients of each batch are summed and the network is updated, even though the batches are randomly chosen each time they're needed. Online SGD selects an element randomly, calculates the gradient and updates the weights, until the error reaches an acceptable level. Randomly choosing elements usually results in faster convergence to an acceptable weight rather than looping through the entire training set.

The basis is now set for the introduction of the weight update method. Equation 2.35 shows the formula to update the weights for backpropagation [33]:

$$\Delta\omega_{(t)} = -\epsilon\frac{\partial E}{\partial \omega_{(t)}} + \alpha\Delta\omega_{(t-1)} \tag{2.35}$$

Essentially, Equation 2.35 calculates the weight update as the product of the gradient (represented by $\frac{\partial E}{\partial \omega_{(t)}}$) and the learning rate (represented by ϵ), while summing the product of the previous changes (represented by $\Delta\omega_{(t-1)}$) and the momentum (represented by α) [33]. The direction of the weight update is inversely related to the gradient's sign (positive gradients should cause a decrease in weight and vice versa, hence the minus signal in 2.35).

Learning Rate

The choice of learning rate and momentum is extremely important to the neural network's performance, and the process of choice is mostly trial and error [33].

Learning rate should not be too high or too low, as the former may cause the network to fail to converge and have a high global error, while the latter maube cause the network to converge extremely slowly. Nevertheless, it should be kept low, as it makes the training more meticulous, while high learning rates might skip past optimal weights [33].

Convolutional Neural Networks

Image features can be categorized into two types: **low-level features** (e.g., lines and dots), and **high-level features**, which are built upon the latter. Convolutional Neural Networks perform a hierarchical construction of an input image: earlier layers process the low-level features from the input images, and deeper layers build more complex structures (i.e., high-level features) based on the low-level features [40].

The most commonly used network architecture is the **LeNET-5** (LeCun et al, 1998). This architecture is illustrated in Figure 2.15-

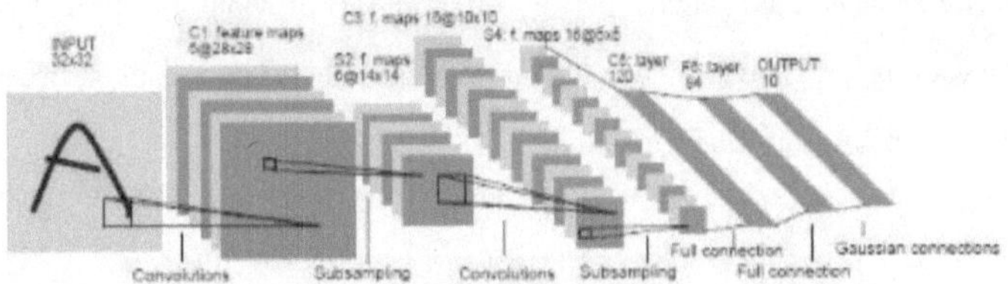

Figure 2.15: LeNET-5 neural network [33]

It also benefits from the backpropagation algorithm discussed in the previous section. Many other network architectures exist (3D-Unet, AlexNet, VGG), however the LeNET-5 architecture laid down the basis for the development of more advanced networks. It is composed of three types of neuron layers [33]:

- Convolutional layers;

- Max-pool layers;

- Dense layers.

Dropout layers are a common and modern addition to Convolutional Neural Network (CNN) architectures and not only help augment their performance, but also reduce overfitting; however, this last layer type will be discussed in the following section.

Convolutional layers' main purpose is to detect images features with the help of **filters** (square-shaped objects that scan over an image). Images are digitally represented by matrices (3 for RGB images and 1 for grayscale images), therefore a filter can be thought of as a grid that sweeps left to right over each matrix row [33]. This neuron layer has the following hyperparameters [33]:

- Number of filters;

- Filter size;

- Stride;

- Padding;

- Activation function.

A convolutional layer has weights between it and the previous layer, and set weights for each pixel on each layer, therefore the number of weights between a convolutional layer and its predecessor is given by Equation 2.36 [33]:

$$[Filter size] \times [Filter size] \times [Number of filters] \tag{2.36}$$

The padding refers to the number of borders of zeros the image will have, while the stride is the step at which the filter will pass through the input image. Figure 2.16 shows the example of a padded image with its strided filter.

0	0	0	0	0	0	0	0	0	0
0	1	3	2	8	4	2	1	3	0
0	0	5	4	8	7	3	2	1	0
0	8	1	8	4	1	3	6	2	0
0	18	4	8	1	23	2	4	17	0
0	19	8	24	14	22	10	11	12	0
0	20	62	23	9	21	6	7	4	0
0	3	13	17	5	13	16	2	8	0
0	0	0	0	0	0	0	0	0	0

Figure 2.16: Convolutional filter with a size of 4 and padding of 1 [33]

Essentially, the filter must start at the top-left border, move for a certain number of steps and end at the bottom-right border. Equation 2.37 shows the number of steps a convolutional filter must take in order to cross an entire image [33]:

$$steps = \frac{w - f + 2p}{s + 1} \tag{2.37}$$

where **p** is the padding number, **f** is the filter width, **w** is the image width and **s** is the stride.

If the input to a convolutional layer is another layer of the same type, then the volume's dimensions will be dictated by the layer's hyperparameters. The same holds true for the output of a convolutional layer: the width and height are equal to the filter size; however, the depth will be equal to the number of filters [33].

Max-pool layers downsample the input into smaller dimensions, and progressively decrease the dimensions of the volumes that pass through them, which can help to avoid overfitting. These layers usually come after a convolutional layer, as Figure 2.15 shows. Max-pool layers do not have weights or padding, and the width of the output volume of a max-pool layer is given by Equation 2.38 [33]:

$$w_2 = \frac{w_1 - f}{s + 1} \tag{2.38}$$

where **f** is the **spatial extent** (i.e., the numbers of positions covered by the pooling filter) and **s** is the stride (both hyperparameters of a max-pool layer), w_1 is the previous volume width. The height, given by Equation 2.39, is calculated in a similar manner [33]:

$$h_2 = \frac{h_1 - f}{s + 1} \tag{2.39}$$

where h_1 is the previous height. The depth of the output volume is equal to the input volume. As an example, Figure 2.17 shows a 2×2 pooling operation (f=2 and s=2) in action:

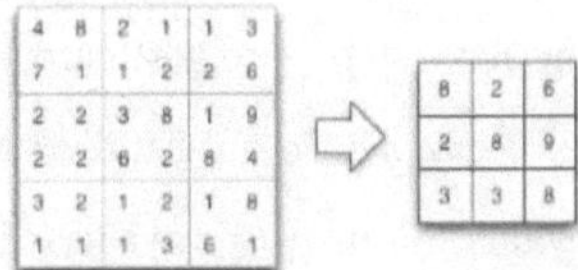

Figure 2.17: Max-pooling example [33]

In Figure 2.17, boxes of 2×2 will be scaled down to single pixels and the highest value of these pixels will represent the 2×2 pixel in the grid.

Dense layers are typically the final layer in this type of neural network and they connect every neuron in the previous layer to each one on the dense layer. The resulting vector is then passed through an activation function (ReLU being the most commonly used). The activation function and number of neurons are the hyperparameters of this layer [33].

Dropout

Dropout works by causing hidden neurons to be unavailable during part of the training, decreasing coadaption between neurons, consequently reducing overfitting [33].

Dropout layers function as a densely connected layer, only that these layers will periodically drop some of their neurons during training. The usual hyperparameters for a dropout layer are [33]:

- **Neuron count:** number of neurons in the dropout layer;

- **Activation function:** choice of function to use in order to format the input;

- **Dropout probability:** likelihood of a neuron dropping out during training.

Dropout works in a similar manner to ensemble modelling. Each network that results from a different set of neurons being dropped out can be thought of as an individual model in an ensemble. More networks will be created as training progresses; however, this new neural network models are temporary. The output is a single network, instead of an ensemble of models to be averaged together [33].

2.3.4 Evaluation

After the models are built, the next step is to estimate their accuracies, as well as their correctly and incorrectly classified examples on unseen data and compare their respective performances. In this section, the evaluation metrics used for this **book** will be explained. Before discussing the various evaluation methods, one will have to explain the concepts of **positive examples** and **negative examples**: the former refers to the examples that belong to the main class of interest (which in this thesis's context is who requires surgery), and the latter refers to the rest of the data [34]. Let P and N be the number of positive and negative examples (respectively); then, for each one of them, the classifier's predicted class is compared to the known class. Every example, after classification, falls into one of the following categories [34]:

- **True Positive (TP):** Correctly labeled positive examples;

- **True Negative (TN):** Correctly labeled negative examples;

- **False Positive (FP):** Negative examples incorrectly labeled as positive;

- **False Negative (FN):** Positive examples incorrectly labeled as negative.

The ground is now layed to the introduction of the evaluation measures used in this **book**.

Confusion Matrix

This performance evaluation method works by showing the user the number of examples the algorithm is classifying correctly (the TP and TN numbers) and incorrectly (the FP and FN numbers), as shown in Table 2.2.

Table 2.2: Confusion Matrix

	surgery not recommended	surgery recommended
does not need surgery	TP	FN
needs surgery	FP	TN

Accuracy

The **accuracy** of a classifier on a given test set is the proportion of test examples correctly labeled by the classifier, i.e. [34]:

$$Accuracy = \frac{TP + TN}{P + N} \tag{2.40}$$

Cross Validation

In **k-fold Cross Validation (CV)**, the initial data are randomly partitioned into k mutually exclusive subsets ("folds") $D_1, D_2, ..., D_k$, each of approximately equal size. Training and test is performed k times. In iteration i, D_i is reserved as the test set, while the remaining partitions are used to train the model. Each sample is used the same number of times for training and once for test. For classification, the accuracy estimate is the overall number of correct classification from the k iterations, divided by the total number of examples in the initial data. **Leave-one-out** is a special case of k-fold CV, where k is set to the number of initial examples, i.e., only one sample is "left out" at a time for the test set [34].

Chapter 3.

State of the art

As it is about to be shown, extensive research on this thesis's topic was done. In this chapter the current knowledge will be analysed, summarized and a critical evaluation will be performed.

3.1 Computer vision in esophageal cancer

The analysis of the literature was based on the publication [17]. A list of the works there reviewed, augmented with other works not considered there, is given in Table 3.1.

Table 3.1: State of the art works (based on [17]). Works with * correspond to binary classification problems.

Paper	Imaging	Goal
[73]	CT	Associate tumour heterogeneity, morphologic tumour response, and Overall Survival (OS)
[11]	CT	Identify patients who develop Radiation Pneumonitis (RP)
[72]	CT	Assess the changes in tumour heterogeneity following neoadjuvant chemotherapy
[63]	CT	Esophagus segmentation
[22]	CT	Esophagus segmentation
[53]	CT	Detection and quantification of local tumor morphological changes due to Chemoradiotherapy (CRT) through Jacobian map

[78]	CT	Evaluation of textural analysis as a prognostic tool in different cancers, including EC
[70]*	CT	Predict Pathological Complete Response (pCR) after neoadjuvant chemoradiotherapy Neoadjuvant Chemotherapy (nCRT) in esophageal squamous cell carcinoma
[6]*	CT + PET	Predict complete response to NCRT
[62]	PET	Study the predictive value of FDG uptake heterogeneity
[61]	PET	Evaluate the reproducibility of texture features
[29]	PET	Risk stratification
[32]	PET	Impact of pre-processing on the quantification of intra-tumour uptake heterogeneity
[19]	PET	Explore the relationship of texture parameters with SUV_{max} and TNM
[58]	PET	Predict pathologic tumour response to CRT
[59]	PET	Predict pathologic tumour response to CRT
[77]*	PET	Prediction of pathologic tumour response
[31]	PET	Investigate the complementary nature of Metabolically Active Tumor Volume (MATV) and texture heterogeneity
[76]	PET	Predict response to neoadjuvant chemotherapy
[35]*	PET	Predict the outcome of a treatment
[36]*	PET	Predict the outcome of a treatment
[75]	PET	Predict response to treatment
[74]	PET	Compare texture features with SUV measures for pathologic response and OS
[56]	PET	Prediction of pCR to CRT before surgery through subjective and quantitative assessement of baseline and postCR FDG-PET

[13]	PET	Predictive and prognostic studies
[48]	PET	Differentiating between FDG-avid Benign Adrenal Tumor (BAT) and Malignant Adrenal Tumor (MAT)
[28]	PET	OS prediction
[47]	PET	Predict tumour response and prognosis
[20]	PET	Effect of smoothing, segmentation, and quantization on heterogeneity measurements
[4]	PET	Improve a radiomics-based model of RP diagnosis in patients undergoing RT
[7]	PET	Assess the value of FDG-PET in predicting PCR to NCRT
[3]*	PET	Evaluate the accuracy of a Three Dimensional Convolutional Neural Network (3D-CNN) feature extraction prediction model
[25]	PET	Usage of FDG-PET-CT scans to describe metabolic nodal stage and response
[69]*	PET	Development of a 3D-CNN prediction model to predict response on esophageal cancer patients

As can be seen, there is no other work that explicitly focus on identifying patients that do not need surgery. There are, however, some works that are closer to the present work in the sense that deal with binary classification problems. Table 3.2 further explores these works by presenting the main methods used and results achieved.

Table 3.2: Binary classification works

Paper	Methods	Results
[70]	55 SCC patients were divied into a training group (44) and test group (11). Logistic regression using Logistic Regression Feature Selection (LRFS) was performed to select predictive clinical parameters and, for radiomic predictors, Least Absolute Shrinkage and Selection Operator (LASSO) along with Logistic Regression (LR) was performed. Only radiomic features were used to build prediction models, since the LR analysis identified no clinical predictors. Furthermore, three LR models were developed to predict pCR and their performances evalutated	Area Under the Receiver Operating Characteristic curve (AUC)s of the developed models were 0.84 to 0.86 (training) and 0.71 to 0.79 (test). There were no differences between them in the training and test groups.
[77]	Four groups of features were examined, recursive feature selection and CV were used for optimal feature selection; SVM and LR models were used for prediction of tumor response to CRT. AUC was used for prediction accuracy measuremente and precision with Confidence Interval (CI)s for the AUC	LR model achieved accuracies of 57%, 73%, 90% and 90%, while SVM achieved 57%, 60%, 94% and 100%.

[35] Feature selection was made using an Evidential Feature Selection (EFS) method and Leave One Out Cross Validation (LOOCV), which were then applied to both esophageal and lung cancer data. Classification was performed using Artificial Neural Network (ANN)s, SVMs and Evidential k-Nearest Neighborhood (EK-NN) (the proposed method). EFS achieved 100% feature selection accuracy and mEK-NN achieved the same value in prediction accuracy.

[36] Feature selection was performed using an improved method discussed in [35]. Classification was also performed using the EK-NN on esophageal, lung and lymph tumor data. Higher robustness and accuracy were observed in the improved EFS method, in all datasets, in comparison to the other methods addressed in the study. Furthermore, the EK-NN also showed higher AUC using the proposed feature selection method, in all data.

[6]	Analysis of clinical, geometric and pre-treatment features extracted from PET and CT data. 6 prediction models using these features as predictors were constructed using Least Absolute Shrinkage (LAS) and Selection Operator Regularization (SOR) logistic regression, and their results were compared to a SUV_{max}-based prediction model. Internal validation was performed to estimate model performance.	AUCs of 0.78 and 0.58 were reported for the 6 prediction models that used the discussed features, and the SUV_{max}-based model (respectively). Using internal validation, the AUCs decreased to 0.74 and 0.54.
[3]	Development of a 3D-CNN prediction model that extracts 3D image features from data, which was used on 97 patients with EC from PET images, and its performance was compared to five other methods across 3 different experiments.	The proposed method outperformed its counterparts in the 3 experiments it was subjected to, achieving accuracies of 83%, 72% and 75% (respectively).
[69]	3D-CNN model based on a ResNet model trained with 798 PET images of SCC and 309 PET images of Lung Cancer (LC). Pretraining with all images was performed to classify them into EC or LC (first stage). 548 PET images (out of 798) were then included in the second stage of classification into survival or expiration one year after diagnosis.	5-year survival rate of 32.6% for patients with expiration of one year after diagnosis, considerably worse than the 50.5% 5-year survival rate for patients predicted to survive and were alive one year after diagnosis.

It can be further noticed that, across all 6 binary classification works on Table 3.2, only [6] combined information from both CT and PET. It is also worth noting that [77] and [36] used spatial-temporal PET features.

3.2 Publicly available databases

A list of publicly available datasets can be found in Table 3.3. To the best of our knowledge, there are no publicly available databases for PET, nor multi-modal datasets comprising both CT and PET as the one used in the present work.

Table 3.3: Publicly available databases [17]

Imaging	Database	Short description	Works
CT	Medical Image Computing and Computer Assisted Intervention Society (MICCAI) 2015 "Synapse" [1]	The focus of the sub-dataset "Abdomen" subdataset is to label 13 abdominal organs, including the esophagus. The sub-dataset consists on a set of 50 abdomen CT scans.	[22]
	The Cancer Genome Atlas Esophageal Carcinoma (TCGA-ESCA) [2]	This dataset is part of a larger effort to build a research community focused on connecting cancer phenotypes to genotypes by providing clinical images matched to subjects from TCGA. The database consists on a set of 17 studies from 16 patients.	-
PET	not found	-	-

---

[1] Available at www.synapse.org

[2] Available at https://wiki.cancerimagingarchive.net/display/Public/TCGA-ESCA

3.3 Discussion

"Traditional" learning algorithms (such as LR, SVM, k-NN and ANNs) offer a relatively good performance in classifying esophageal cancer data, and thus are widely used in biomedical imaging and in the field of computer vision as a whole. One drawback, however, is that they often have to be paired with a feature extraction method before classifying the data, i.e., an additional step in the process.

Deep Learning algorithms, such as CNNs, are also used to process imaging data and not only classify image data but also have the feature extraction capability embedded in them (i.e., they "learn" the features) and their performances have been shown to be close to that of humans [57]. The only drawback is that they need considerable amounts of data in order to have significant test accuracies [15], for which data augmentation is used [76].

Chapter 4.
Material and Methods

In this section, the information about the data will be explored, and the full pipeline of this book will be explained. Special thanks to Doutora Olga Sousa, from the Radioncology department of the Portuguese Institute of Oncology of Porto, for providing the patients' data used in this book.

4.1 Dataset

This data was acquired the context of the ESTIMA project, and a prospective cohort study of consecutively sampled patients allocated to neoadjuvant chemo-radiotherapy (NCRT) regimen according to local protocols was performed. For this particular early stage, curative, resectable disease cohort of patients, the inclusion criteria was diagnosis of squamous cell carcinoma, undifferentiated carcinoma or adenocarcinoma of esophageal or esophagealgastric junction (Siewert I e II) and clinical Stage II or III disease, according to American Joint Committee on Cancer Staging classification, 7th edition.

All patients presented the upper border of the tumor at least 3 cm below the upper esophageal sphincter. All patient signed an informed consent and the study was approved by the institution ethics committee. Exclusion criteria included pregnant or lactating women, previous thoracic radiotherapy, Impaired haematological, hepatic, renal or pulmonary function defined, neutrophils count $< 1.5 \times 10^9/L$, platelet count $< 100 \times 10^9/L$, serum concentration of total bilirubin $> 1.5 \times ULN$ (upper limit of normal range), creatinine $> 120mcmol/L$, FEV1 (Forced expiratory volume in 1 second) $< 1.5L$ and active infection or other medical condition that prevents the patient from receiving the planed treatment.

The study flow diagram can be seen in Figure 4.1. As can be seen, all patients underwent pre-treatment staging and evaluation, which included Computed tomography (CT) of the neck, chest, and upper abdomen and 18F-FDG (fluorodeoxyglucose) Positron Emission Tomography (PET-CT). Patients are then submitted to neoadjuvant radio-chemotherapy and surgery seven weeks after the end of radiation therapy.

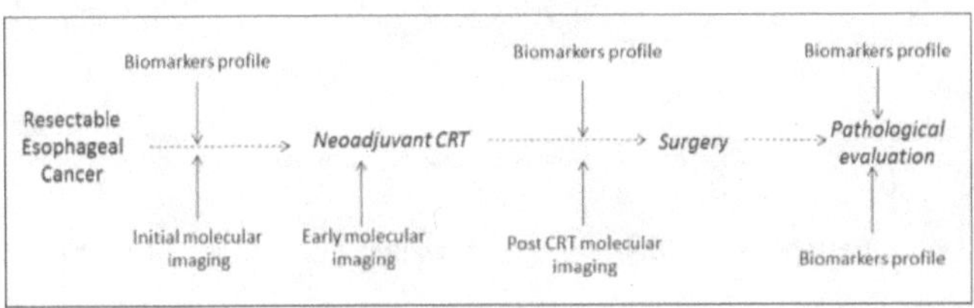

Figure 4.1: Acquisition flow diagram

In summary, molecular imaging (PET/CT) images were acquired at three time points:

- Baseline study: 18-Fluorodeoxyglucose (18-F)-FDG PET/CT performed with a maximum interval of 21 days until the start of CRT;

- Early molecular imaging study: 18-F-FDG PET/CT, performed preferably on the 8th after the start of CRT (before the 2nd chemotherapy cycle);

- Post CRT study: 18-F-FDG PET/CT, performed 6 weeks after CRT.

The assessment of pathologic response was performed using an adaptation of the EURECA CC2 guidelines [64]. The report follows the College of American Pathologist's guidelines, with assessment of the extent of tumor response.

The training database consists of CT, Planned Target Volume (PTV) and PET images (from 14 patients), with a total of 70 images (14 CT + 14 PTV + 42 PET) that follow the ESTIMA protocol. Figure 4.2 shows the number of patients who had incomplete and complete response. CT volumes were acquired with a pixel spacing between 0.9 and 1.6 mm and a difference of patient position between adjacent slices between 2.5 and 5.0 mm, all in the DICOM format. PET images from 14 patients were acquired (3 for each patient), also in the DICOM format, with a pixel spacing of 4.0 mm and with a slice thickness between 3.0 and 4.0 mm.

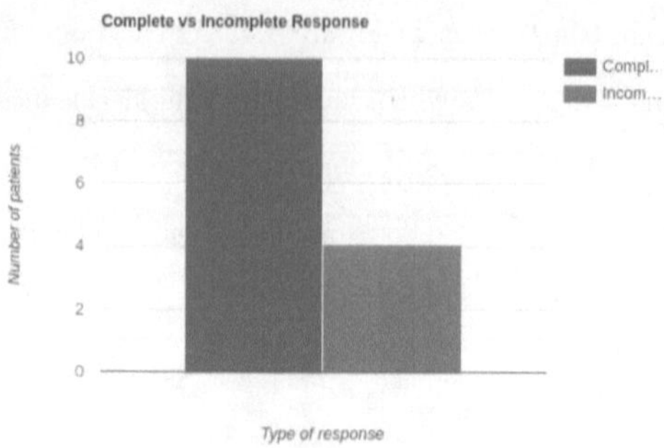

Figure 4.2: Complete vs Incomplete response

An example of a patient for which surgery was necessary is given in Figure 4.3; while an example of a patient that did not need to have surgery is given in Figure 4.4.

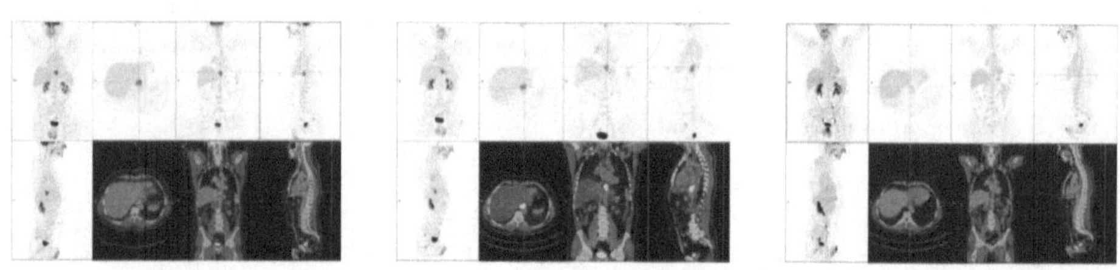

(a) Baseline   (b) Early molecular imaging   (c) Post CRT

Figure 4.3: Example of a patient with complete pathological response

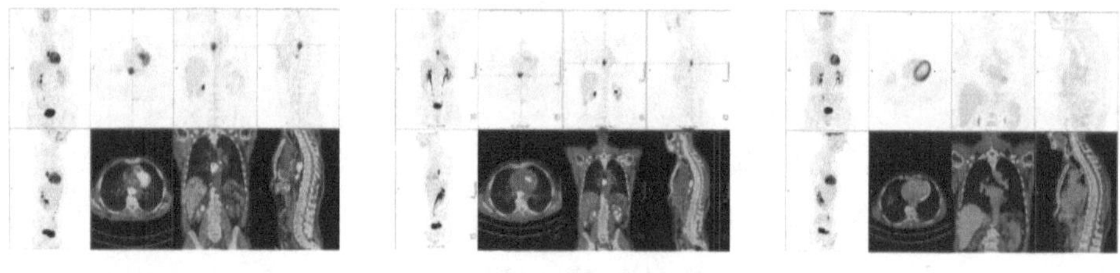

(a) Baseline   (b) Early molecular imaging   (c) Post CRT

Figure 4.4: Example of a patient with incomplete pathological response

4.2 Image Pre-processing

In this section, the pre-processing of the images used for this book will be discussed, as well as the full pipeline of this work.

4.2.1 Image Rescaling and Rotation

CT and PET images from the dataset suffered from different scaling and orientation issues, by which all images were resampled to a voxel size 4x4x4 and then, for the PET images, two rotations of 90 degrees anticlockwise on both the Y-axis and Z-axis. One of the patients' PET/CT images needed an additional 180 degress clockwise on the Z-axis, for it was necessary for it to be on the same orientation as its CT counterpart, as shown by Figure 4.5.

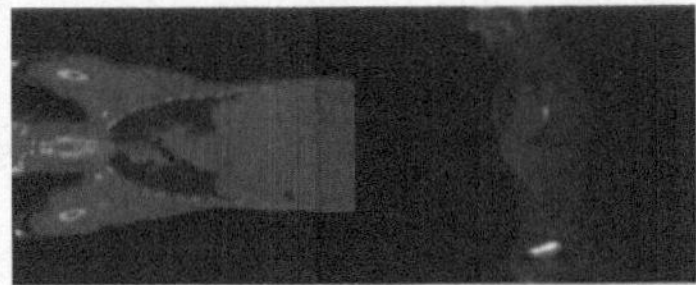 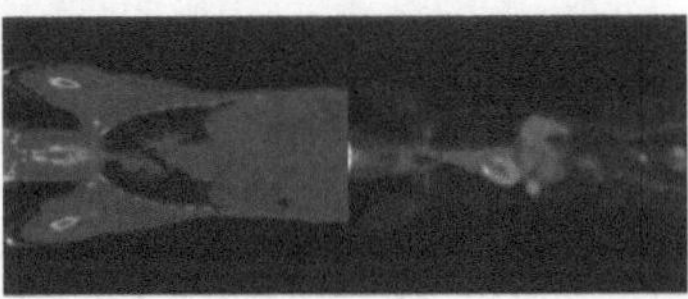

Figure 4.5: Example of an image rotation applied to the dataset. The first picture shows the original images, whilst the second one shows that both images are now in the same orientation. For illustrative purposes, only one slice per modality was used.

4.2.2 Co-registration

The PTV segmentation was manually performed in CT. This information needs thus to be translated into the PET data. Here, the technique proposed in [51] is used. It was carried out by selecting the CT volumes as a reference and then aligning all PET data with the former so that both volumes overlap with each other. Figure 4.6 shows an example of co-registration on images for the dataset in question.

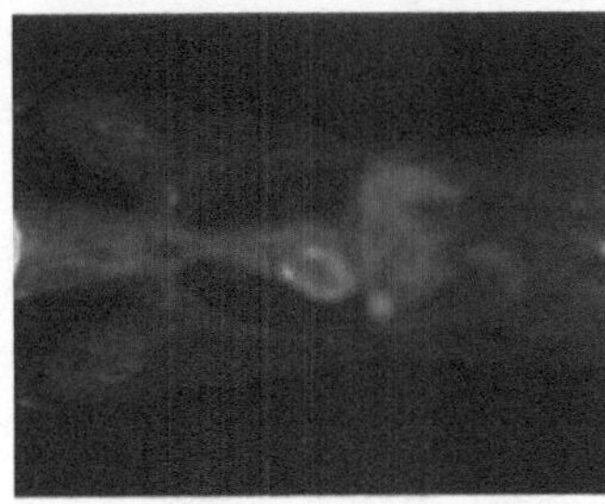

Figure 4.6: Co-registration of CT and PET volumes

4.3 Experimental Setup

The software MATrix LABoratory (MATLAB) was used for the work in this book, and the Leave-one-out Cross Validation method of evaluation was performed on all experiments. Precision and confusion matrices were used to evaluate the accuracy of the methods.

4.4 Full pipeline

Figure 4.7 shows the full pipeline for this work. After the data is collected, it goes through a validation phase, where every PET and CT image is rotated, in order to have the same orientation; then, their voxel sizes are validated and both images are co-registered. Finally, they are subjected to traditional and deep learning algorithms for classification:

- **Traditional Pipeline:** the images' features are extracted through the use of *regionprops3*, and then are selected using feature selection algorithms, in order to be classified using traditional classifiers;

- **Deep Learning Pipeline:** the images' features are extracted using pretrained networks, as well as trained from scratch ones. Then, they go through two different phases:

  - **Traditional classification:** after extraction, the features are then classified using traditional classifiers;

  - **Full Deep Learning classification:** after extraction, the features are classified using CNNs.

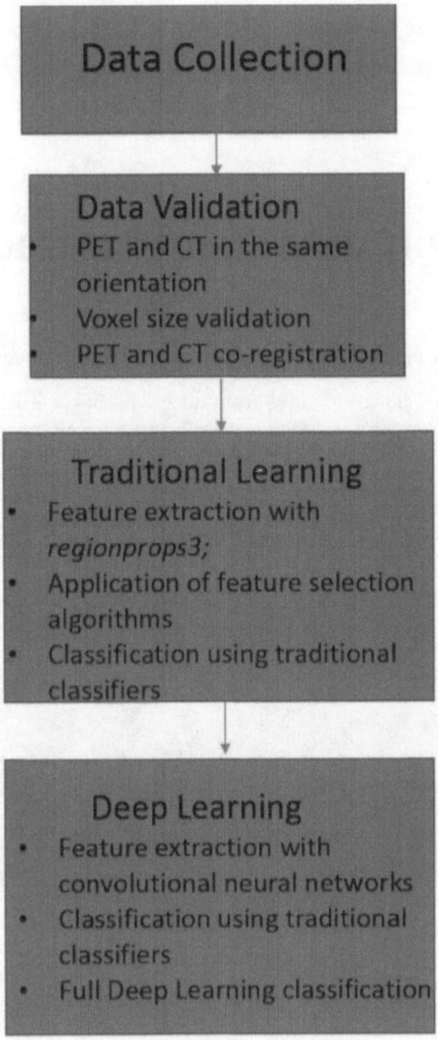

Figure 4.7: Full Pipeline for this work

Chapter 5.

Classification with hand-crafted features

The first classification method that is going to be performed on our data is the hand-crafted features method. Firstly, image features from all modalities will be extracted then classified using the classifiers introduced in section 2.3.1. Then, feature selection algorithms will be applied to the fused features, for further classification. Lastly, decision fusion on the outputs of the classifiers will be performed, by majority voting and average voting. Figure 5.1 illustrates the steps the data will go through in this stage.

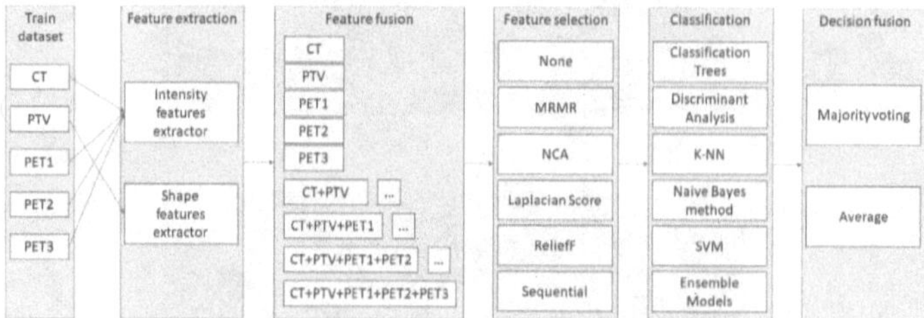

Figure 5.1: Hand-Crafted Features Classification pipeline

5.1 Feature extraction

MATLAB's *regionprops3* function was used for feature extraction, which was performed by first applying it to the PTV image, which is a binary volume, and then using it alongside the PTV and PET data. A list of possible features that can be extracted from Three-dimensional (3D) volumes is given in Table 5.3.

Table 5.1: 3D images features

	Feature	Description
Shape Measurements	Bounding Box	Smallest cuboid containing the region
	Centroid	Center of mass of the region
	Convex Hull	Smallest convex polygon that can contain the region
	Convex Image	Image of the convex hull
	Convex Volume	Number of voxels in the Convex Image
	Eigenvalues	Eigenvalues of the voxels representing a region
	Eigenvectors	Eigenvectors of the voxels representing a region
	EquivDiameter	Diameter of a sphere with the same volume as the region
	Extent	Ratio of voxels in the region to voxels in the total bounding box
	Image	Bounding box of the region
	Orientation	Euler angles
	Principal Axis Length	Length (in voxels) of the major axes of the ellipsoid that have the same normalized second central moments as the region
	Solidity	Proportion of the voxels in the convex hull that are also in the region
	Subarray Index	Indices used to extract elements inside the object bounding box
	Surface Area	Distance around the boundary of the region

	Volume	Count of the actual number of 'on' voxels in the region
	Voxel Index List	Linear indices of the voxels in the region
	Voxel List	Locations of voxels in the region
Voxel Value Measurements	Max Intensity	Value of the voxel with the greatest intensity in the region
	Mean Intensity	Mean of all the intensity values in the region
	Min Intensity	Value of the voxel with the lowest intensity in the region
	Voxel Values	Value of the voxels in the region
	Weighted Centroid	Center of the region based on location and intensity value

5.2 Classifiers

The classifiers used for the traditional method of classification were Classification Trees, Discriminant Analysis, K-NN, Naive Bayes method, Support Vector Machines and Ensemble Models.

5.3 Fusion

Fusion can be performed at different levels. Two possible examples of fusion are fusion at feature level (where features are, for instance, concatenated), and at decision level (for instance by voting or averaging the results of the individual classifiers). Both feature level and decision level fusion will be applied in this section and results from both methods will be compared.

5.4 Results

In Table 5.2 are the reported accuracies for classification using the classifiers discussed in Section 2.3.1 and listed in Section 5.2 for completeness.

It can be noticed that Discriminant Analysis classifier yielded the best results of all its counterparts, as it achieved accuracies higher than 50% on all image modalities, even though it underperformed in CT and PET images, relatively to the PTV.

The SVM and Naive Bayes also performed well, achieving higher or equal to 50% accuracies on all modalities. The K-NN classifier underperformed only on CT, achieving an accuracy of 42.86%. However, the SVM had the highest accuracy on CT, whereas Naive Bayes and K-NN performed considerably better than SVM on the rest of the data. The Classification Ensembles model also performed well, underperforming only on the PTV, with an accuracy of $\approx 28.57\%$.

Classification Trees had the worst performance of all 7 classifiers, achieving lower than 50% on all modalities except CT, where it achieved 50%. The Classification Tree Ensemble model performed well on the PTV and CT modalities, however it underperformed on the PET scans.

Table 5.2: Accuracy (%) of each method used on the hand-crafted features. In bold are the best accuracies for each image type.

	PTV	CT	PET1	PET2	PET3
Classification Trees	35.71	50.00	42.86	42.86	42.86
Discriminant Analysis	**92.86**	64.29	57.14	57.14	57.14
k-Nearest Neighbors	57.14	42.86	**64.29**	**64.29**	**64.29**
Naive Bayes	57.14	64.29	**64.29**	**64.29**	**64.29**
SVM	50.00	**71.43**	50.00	50.00	50.00
Classification Ensembles	28.57	57.14	57.14	57.14	57.14
Classification Tree Ensembles	64.29	**71.43**	35.71	42.86	42.86

With the exception of Discriminant Analysis (with an accuracy of 92.86%), the accuracies of the methods used were considerably low, which may be due to the small number of data used.

As pointed out in Section 5.3, fusion was first performed at feature level, i.e., features from the PTV, CT and the three PET scans were concatenated. All of the combinations were attempted, meaning that 31 possible feature combinations were analyzed and classified using the 7 classifiers in 5.2, with a total of 217 (31 feature combinations $\times$ 7 classifiers) classifications performed. To keep the document contained, only the maximum accuracies for each classifier are shown. The results are summarized in Tables 5.3 and 5.4.

Both the Discriminant Analysis and Support Vector Machine classifiers reached accuracies of 92.86% and 71.43% whilst using features from PTV and CT (respectively).

Table 5.3: Best accuracies (%) of the first 5 classifiers, with each respective feature set(s) for each one. The '+' sign denotes the combination between the features of each image modality.

	Accuracy (%)	Feature sets
Classification Trees	57.14	PTV+CT
		PTV+CT+PET1
		PTV+CT+PET2
		PTV+CT+PET3
		PTV+CT+PET1+PET2
		PTV+CT+PET1+PET3
		PTV+CT+PET2+PET3
		PTV+CT+PET1+PET2+PET3
Discriminant Analysis	92.86	PTV
k-Nearest Neighbors	64.29	PET1, PET2, PET3
		PET1+PET2
		PET1+PET3
		PET2+PET3
		PET1+PET2+PET3
Naive Bayes	64.29	CT
		PET1, PET2, PET3
		PET1+PET2
		PET1+PET3
		PET2+PET3
		PET1+PET2+PET3
Support Vector Machine	71.43	CT

Table 5.4: Best accuracies (%) for the last 2 classifiers, with each respective feature set(s) for each one. The '+' sign denotes the combination between the features of each image modality.

	Accuracy (%)	Feature sets
Classification Ensemble	57.14	CT
		PET1, PET2, PET3
		PET1+PET2
		PET1+PET3
		PET2+PET3
		PET1+PET2+PET3
		PTV+CT
		PTV+CT+PET1
		PTV+CT+PET2
		PTV+CT+PET3
		PTV+CT+PET1+PET2
		PTV+CT+PET1+PET3
		PTV+CT+PET2+PET3
		PTV+CT+PET1+PET2+PET3
Classification Tree Ensembles	64.29	CT+PET1
		CT+PET2
		CT+PET2+PET3
		CT+PET1+PET2+PET3

By combining PTV and CT features with all of the PET data, the Classification Trees classifier had an accuracy of 57.14%, the same as the Classification Ensemble, only that the latter used CT features separately and PET data both separately and combined.

The k-Nearest Neighbors and Naive Bayes classifiers reached accuracies of 64.29%, using all the PET data and the CT features (for the NB classifier). The Classification Tree Ensemble model had similar performance, albeit using CT and PET features simultaneously.

As mentioned in section 5.3, decision level fusion was also performed, albeit with less satisfying results.

Firstly, the various image modalities were adequately classified using the classifiers that yielded the best results for each one of them:

- **PTV:** Discriminant Analysis;

- **CT:** Support Vector Machine;

- **PET1, PET2 and PET3:** Naive Bayes.

The labels for each image modality were then gathered together and that is where voting was used. Two types of voting were used:

- **Voting by mean:** The mean of the labels is taken as the predicted class;

- **Voting by mode:** The mode of the labels (i.e., the most frequent label) is the predicted class.

The true classes were then compared to each one of the outputs of the methods described above, with both of them achieving accuracies of 64.29%.

As for the feature selection, the NCA, ReliefF and Sequential Feature Selection produced the following results:

- **Neighborhood Component Analysis:** using the *Orientation (yaw)*, *Surface Area* and *Volume* as predictors, this filter type algorithm performed well on the Classification Trees, Naive Bayes and Classification Tree Ensembles models, with accuracies of 71.43%, 50% and 64.24%. However, it underperformed on K-NN, with an accuracy of 42.86% Discriminant Analysis and SVM got 35.71% accuracies and Classification Ensemble had 28.57%, with the latter being the worst performance.

- **ReliefF:** this filter type algorithm used the second and third *Eigenvalues, Orientation (roll)* and *Bounding Box's* z coordinate as predictors. It had 50% accuracies on the Discriminant Analysis, Classification Ensembles and Classification Tree Ensembles models, whereas it underperformed on the SVM, with an accuracy of 35.71%, and on the Classification Trees, K-NN and Naive Bayes models, with accuracies of 28.57%.

- **Sequential Feature Selection:** Using the *Bounding Box*'s x coordinate and the first *Eigenvalue*, Wrapper Type feature selection proved to be the most effective, as the SVM and K-NN boasted accuracies of 92.86% and 85.71% (respectively). The Classification Trees (both single and Ensemble) and Discriminant Analysis classifiers performed at 64.29%, and the lowest performances came from the Naive Bayes and Classification Ensembles, with 57.14% and 50% accuracies (respectively).

Tables 5.5 and 5.6 show the confusion matrix of the SVM and K-NN models for the Wrapper Type feature selection method. For this particular problem, it would be worse to not perform sugery on a patient who needs it, than to perform surgery on a patient who does not need it.

Table 5.5: Confusion matrix for the SVM model

	surgery not recommended	surgery recommended
does not need surgery	9	0
needs surgery	1	4

As it can be seen, the SVM model captured only one false positive with the sequential feature algorithm, i.e., it did not recommend surgery to a patient who needs it. As for the K-NN model, it had two false positives, as it can be seen on Table 5.6. Therefore, the SVM model can be considered the best traditional model.

Table 5.6: Confusion matrix for the K-NN model

	surgery not recommended	surgery recommended
does not need surgery	9	0
needs surgery	2	3

Illustrative results of correctly and incorrectly classified cases are given in Figure 5.2. It is clear the similarity between the PTV of the two cases that were recommended by the SVM not to perform surgery, although the patient on the left did not needed surgery, but the patient on the middle did needed it and was thus incorrectly classified.

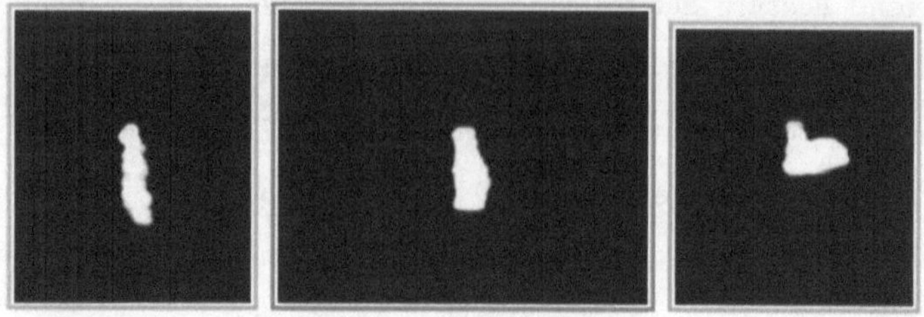

Figure 5.2: Best traditional model results (only the slice with the biggest PTV area is shown). Left: Correctly classified patient that does not need surgery; Middle: Incorrectly classified patient that needs surgery; Right: Correctly classified patient that needs surgery.

5.5 Conclusions

Selected best results for the traditional learning method can be seen in Table 5.7. It can be seen that the PTV data seems to convey important information to discriminate patients that need surgery from the ones that do not. It can also be seen that single modality training offers the best results in comparison with the fusion methods (feature and decision level).

Table 5.7: Traditional Learning selected results. In bold are the best accuracies.

Imaging	Feature selection	Classifier	Accuracy (%)
PTV	none	DA	**92.86**
CT	none	SVM	71.43
CT	none	CTE	71.43
PET1	none	kNN	64.29
PET1	none	NB	64.29
PET2	none	kNN	64.29
PET2	none	NB	64.29
PET3	none	kNN	64.29
PET3	none	NB	64.29
PTV	Sequential	SVM	**92.86**

Moreover, feature selection does not seem to be able to improve these results, as the classifier with only two features chosen by Sequential feature selection, was able to achieve the same results as the classifier with the full set of features.

Chapter 6.

Classification with learnt features

In the last section, traditional learning techniques in the context of this work were explored, to varying but overall satisfying degrees of accuracy. In this section, deep learning techniques, such as **transfer learning** will be explored. Similarly to the previous section, leave one out cross validation was used for the evaluation of the neural networks' performance.

For this method, the slice with the biggest PTV area was manually identified. Then, that slice, the previous one and the one after were retrieved to form 2D images with 3 channels. Examples retrieved from two patients are given in Figure 6.1.

Data augmentation was performed on the training images: the images were rotated 45 degrees, both anticlockwise and clockwise, reflections (in the x axis) and translations of 30 pixels were also applied; moreover, the data also suffered scaling operations, to 90% and 110% of their original size. Training was endured with Adam optimizer, using a batch size of one, six maximum epochs, and an initial learning rate of 3×10^{-4}.

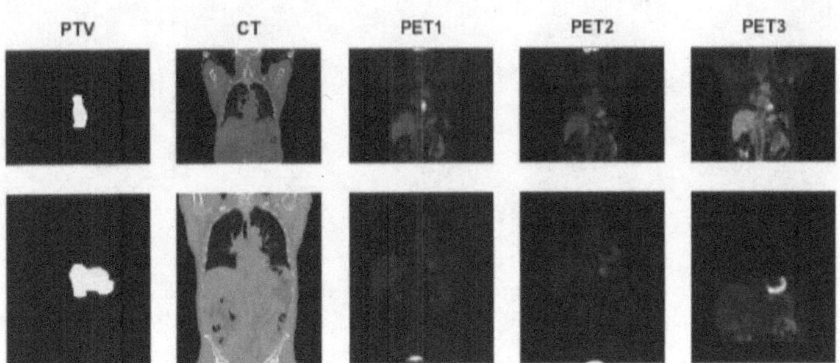

Figure 6.1: Selected slices from two patients

6.1 Deep learning for feature extraction

In this section, image features will not be manually extracted from the data, **transfer learning** will be used instead.

Transfer learning consists in utilizing the pretrained weights of a certain network on a different problem. Pretrained CNNs were used in this context, which in turn will "learn" the features that will be used for image classification. The features were extracted using five different neural network architectures: *Resnet-101, Inception-ResNet-v2, AlexNet, VGG-16* and *VGG-19*. The three latter networks follow practically the same structure, i.e., all of them have convolutional, ReLU and pooling layers one after the other, and the complexity increases from the AlexNet (least complex) to the VGG-19 (most complex). As for the *ResNet101* and *InceptionResNetv2* architectures, these are considerably more complex than the remaining three, as both possess multiple parallel layers for further data processing. Visual representations of these architectures can be seen on appendix A.

Moreover, both low-level and high-level features were extracted from the neural network algorithms and were classified using the same classifiers as traditional learning. The full pipeline can be seen in Figure 6.2. An example of low and high level feature extraction on the *VGG-16* network can also be seen in Figure 6.3

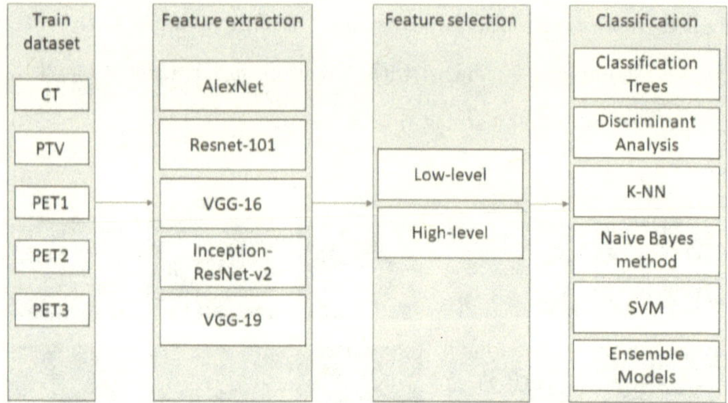

Figure 6.2: Deep Learning for feature extraction (transfer learning)

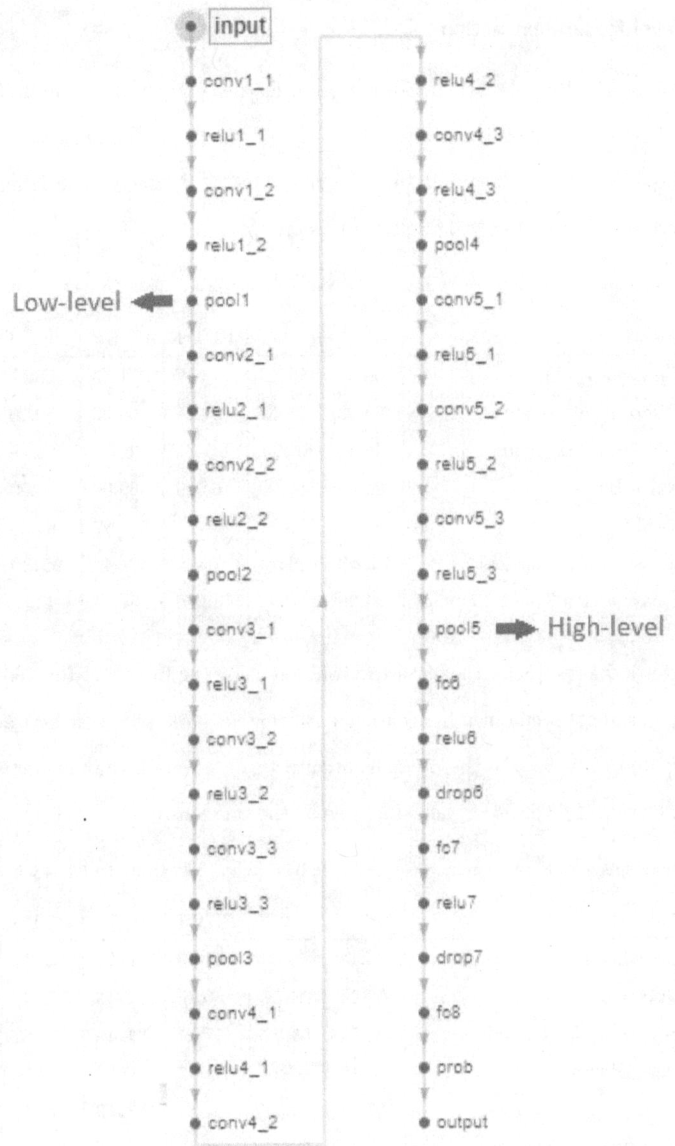

Figure 6.3: Illustration of High and Low level features on VGG-16 network.

6.1.1 High-level feature extraction

Table 6.1 shows the Resnet-101's performance on feature extraction of the data. It can be seen that the best results for this network architecture come from combining the Classification Ensembles classifier with the PET3 data, achieving 92.86% accuracy. The remaining data's accuracies were between 71.43% (the worst in this group) and 85.71%.

Table 6.1: Resnet-101 accuracy (%) results. In bold are the best accuracies for each image type.

Algorithm	PTV	CT	PET 1	PET 2	PET 3
Classification Trees	50.00	71.43	78.57	71.43	78.57
Discriminant Analysis	64.29	78.57	57.14	64.29	50.00
k-Nearest Neighbours	42.86	**85.71**	**85.71**	**78.57**	64.29
Naive Bayes	21.43	50.00	64.29	50.00	50.00
SVM	57.14	78.57	**85.71**	**78.57**	64.29
Classification Ensembles	**71.43**	71.43	78.57	71.43	**92.86**
Classification Tree Ensembles	64.29	50.00	42.86	57.14	42.86

In Table 6.2 are the results for the feature extraction using the Inception-ResNet-v2 architecture. There was a slight step down in accuracy with this network, as the highest accuracy was 85.71% (compared to 92.86% of the previous architecture). Overall, the remaining accuracies were in the interval [71.43,85.71]%, i.e., the same as the previous model.

Table 6.2: Inception-ResNet-v2 accuracy (%) results. In bold are the best accuracies for each image type.

Algorithm	PTV	CT	PET 1	PET 2	PET 3
Classification Trees	57.14	71.43	71.43	35.71	**85.71**
Discriminant Analysis	57.14	**78.57**	50.00	**71.43**	71.43
k-Nearest Neighbours	35.71	**78.57**	57.14	**71.43**	78.57
Naive Bayes	**71.43**	57.14	**78.57**	57.14	57.14
SVM	57.14	**78.57**	57.14	**71.43**	71.43
Classification Ensembles	50.00	71.43	71.43	42.86	**85.71**
Classification Tree Ensembles	50.00	71.43	57.14	57.14	64.29

Table 6.3 shows the performance of the classifiers on the features extracted with the VGG-16 network architecture. There was a considerable increase in accuracy, as the Classification Ensembles model achieved 100% accuracy, paired with the CT data, while the remaining classifiers

also stayed in the [71.43,85.71] accuracy range.

Table 6.3: VGG-16 accuracy (%) results. In bold are the best accuracies for each image type.

Algorithm	PTV	CT	PET 1	PET 2	PET 3
Classification Trees	**85.71**	78.57	64.29	21.43	71.43
Discriminant Analysis	64.29	85.71	**78.57**	**71.43**	**78.57**
k-Nearest Neighbours	64.29	85.71	71.43	50.00	71.43
Naive Bayes	50.00	71.43	57.14	28.57	42.86
SVM	57.14	85.71	71.43	50.00	71.43
Classification Ensembles	71.43	**100.00**	64.29	42.86	71.43
Classification Tree Ensembles	57.14	64.29	50.00	42.86	50.00

Table 6.4 shows the results for the VGG-19 architecture. The Discriminant Analysis classifier achieved the highest accuracy on the high-level extraction method, on the PET1 images, while the remaining classifiers achieved accuracies in the [71.43,78.57] range.

Table 6.4: VGG-19 accuracy (%) results. In bold are the best accuracies for each image type.

Algorithm	PTV	CT	PET 1	PET 2	PET 3
Classification Trees	35.71	42.86	78.57	21.43	57.14
Discriminant Analysis	**78.57**	71.43	**92.86**	64.29	**78.57**
k-Nearest Neighbours	50.00	**78.57**	64.29	57.14	50.00
Naive Bayes	42.86	57.14	85.71	50.00	71.43
SVM	57.14	**78.57**	71.43	50.00	64.29
Classification Ensembles	50.00	50.00	78.57	57.14	57.14
Classification Tree Ensembles	42.86	64.29	71.43	**71.43**	50.00

Finally, Table 6.5 shows the results for the Alexnet architecture. The CT data boast the bigger number of highest accuracies with this network architecture, achieving 92.86% with the K-NN, SVM and Classification Tree Ensembles, while the remaining classifiers stayed in the [64.29,85.71]% range.

In conclusion, it can be noticed that less complex network architectures like the *AlexNet* and *VGG-16* yield better results, in comparison to the more complex *ResNet101* and *InceptionRes-Netv2*.

Table 6.5: AlexNet accuracy (%) results. In bold are the best accuracies for each image type.

Algorithm	PTV	CT	PET 1	PET 2	PET 3
Classification Trees	**64.29**	85.71	71.43	35.71	71.43
Discriminant Analysis	21.43	85.71	**85.71**	**64.29**	**78.57**
k-Nearest Neighbours	35.71	**92.86**	57.14	57.14	42.86
Naive Bayes	35.71	71.43	28.57	42.86	64.29
SVM	35.71	**92.86**	71.43	**64.29**	71.43
Classification Ensembles	28.57	85.71	78.57	35.71	71.43
Classification Tree Ensembles	50.00	**92.86**	64.29	50.00	64.29

6.1.2 Low-level feature extraction

Table 6.6 shows the performance of low-level feature extraction on the ResNet101 network architecture. It can be noticed that the accuracies for the ResNet architecture on low-level features were a considerable step down in comparison to its high-level counterpart, as the highest accuracies were 85.71 (CT+Discriminant Analysis and PET1+Classification Trees).

Table 6.6: Resnet-101 low-level feature extraction results. In bold are the best accuracies (%) for each image type.

Algorithm	PTV	CT	PET 1	PET 2	PET 3
Classification Trees	28.57	64.29	**85.71**	64.29	71.43
Discriminant Analysis	50.00	57.14	50.00	**78.57**	57.14
k-Nearest Neighbours	42.86	**85.71**	64.29	**78.57**	71.43
Naive Bayes	35.71	64.29	78.57	**78.57**	64.29
SVM	**64.29**	64.29	64.29	64.29	64.29
Classification Ensembles	42.86	64.29	78.57	**78.57**	71.43
Classification Tree Ensembles	28.57	50.00	64.29	50.00	**85.71**

As for the Inception-ResNet-v2 (Table 6.7), a similar trend can be noticed, as all the best accuracies for each data were 78.57, which is also a considerable step down in relation to the high-level feature extraction

Algorithm	PTV	CT	PET 1	PET 2	PET 3
Classification Trees	21.43	**78.57**	57.14	50.00	71.43
Discriminant Analysis	**78.57**	64.29	**78.57**	**78.57**	**78.57**
k-Nearest Neighbours	28.57	71.43	71.43	**78.57**	71.43
Naive Bayes	50.00	71.43	71.43	71.43	71.43
SVM	64.29	64.29	64.29	64.29	64.29
Classification Ensembles	42.86	64.29	28.57	71.43	57.14
Classification Tree Ensembles	42.86	64.29	71.43	57.14	57.14

Low-level feature extraction on the VGG-16 network (Table 6.8) shows perhaps the biggest step down in accuracy so far, as the highest accuracy was 85.71% (PET2+Discriminant Analysis), in comparison to the 100% achieved in the high-level method.

Algorithm	PTV	CT	PET 1	PET 2	PET 3
Classification Trees	**64.29**	**78.57**	50.00	42.86	**78.57**
Discriminant Analysis	42.86	64.29	64.29	**85.71**	64.29
k-Nearest Neighbours	42.86	**78.57**	50.00	78.57	71.43
Naive Bayes	57.14	64.29	**78.57**	71.43	64.29
SVM	57.14	71.43	71.43	64.29	**78.57**
Classification Ensembles	28.57	50.00	50.00	57.14	64.29
Classification Tree Ensembles	35.71	50.00	**78.57**	64.29	71.43

The VGG-19 network (Table 6.9) had a roughly similar performance of its high-level counterpart, as the highest accuracy was also 92.86%, even though it registered an accuracy of 50% with the PTV data combined with the Classification Trees classifier.

Table 6.9: VGG-19 low-level feature extraction accuracy (%) results. In bold are the best accuracies for each image type.

Algorithm	PTV	CT	PET 1	PET 2	PET 3
Classification Trees	14.29	35.71	64.29	35.71	64.29
Discriminant Analysis	**50.00**	64.29	64.29	**85.71**	57.14
k-Nearest Neighbours	42.86	**92.86**	57.14	78.57	64.29
Naive Bayes	42.86	78.57	**71.43**	57.14	64.29
SVM	42.86	78.57	57.14	78.57	**78.57**
Classification Ensembles	21.43	57.14	64.29	64.29	71.43
Classification Tree Ensembles	42.86	57.14	50.00	64.29	**78.57**

Lastly, Table 6.10 shows the results for the low-level feature extraction on the AlexNet network architecture. Even though the highest accuracies were equal, the high-level method boasted a higher number of equally high accuracies than the low-level feature extraction method (3 classifiers with 92.86% vs 1 on the low-level method).

Table 6.10: AlexNet low-level feature extraction accuracy (%) results. In bold are the best accuracies for each image type.

Algorithm	PTV	CT	PET 1	PET 2	PET 3
Classification Trees	35.71	78.57	78.57	**85.71**	42.86
Discriminant Analysis	42.86	50.00	64.29	50.00	71.43
k-Nearest Neighbors	**64.29**	57.14	50.00	78.57	64.29
Naive Bayes	28.57	50.00	71.43	64.29	57.14
SVM	**64.29**	85.71	92.86	64.29	**85.71**
Classification Ensembles	57.14	71.43	57.14	57.14	64.29
Classification Tree Ensembles	50.00	57.14	42.86	**85.71**	71.43

A similar trend can be observed in regards to the previous section: network architectures like the *AlexNet*, *VGG-16* and *VGG-19* yielded higher accuracies than their more complex counterparts, even though the accuracies were generally lower than those of the previous section.

6.2 Pre-trained Networks for Classification

In this section, the same five network architectures were used for the classification of the images in question. However, instead of using "traditional learning" classifiers, the five previous network architectures were used not only to "learn" the features but also to classify them. The pipeline is given in Figure 6.4

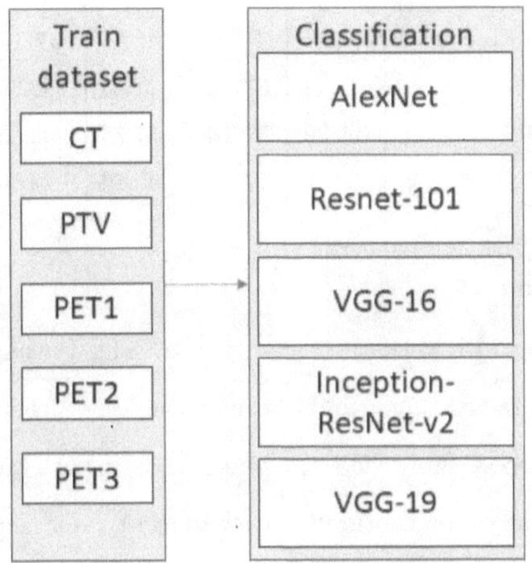

Figure 6.4: Deep Learning for classification (transfer learning)

6.2.1 Single modality training

The original network architectures were designed to run on an images dataset which had 1000 classes [41], therefore the neural networks had to be adapted to this context: the fully connected and output layers were replaced by two other layers with only two neurons, corresponding to the total number of classes of this problem.

The results for the pre-trained network classification method can be seen in Table 6.11. It can be seen that the results for the transfer learning method decreased substantially in quality, as none of the networks in the list above got scores above 78.57%, which in comparison to the previous section is a considerable step down in terms of accuracy.

All of the classifiers in this section underperformed in at least one image modality, with the VGG-19 being the worst offender, as it scored 42.86% in all the PET data. The Inception-ResNet-v2 and VGG-16 all had low performances on two modalities, while the Resnet101 and Alexnet architectures only had accuracies lower than 50.00% on the PET2 data.

Table 6.11: Pre-trained networks classification accuracy (%) results. In bold are the best accuracies for each image type.

Algorithm	PTV	CT	PET 1	PET 2	PET 3
Alexnet	50.00	57.14	**78.57**	42.86	57.14
Inception-ResNet-v2	35.71	50.00	42.86	**57.14**	**64.29**
VGG-16	35.71	**57.14**	71.43	42.86	50.00
Resnet101	**64.29**	**57.14**	57.14	42.86	50.00
VGG-19	50.00	**57.14**	42.86	42.86	42.86

6.2.2 Feature level fusion

Feature level fusion was also performed alongside transfer learning. Ten experiments were carried out, in total, and their results can be seen on Table 6.12. For this part, contrary to the single modality image processing method, the best slice from each image modality was selected and fused in the same images, by considering each image type in a channel.

It can be noticed that the accuracies for each group of data were a considerable step-down in accuracy, comparatively to the previous methods, as the highest accuracy was that of the VGG-16 architecture with the combined features of PTV, CT and PET2 images, while the remaining architectures had equal performances of 64.29% on the PTV, PET2 and PET3 data (Alexnet), the CT, PET2 and PET3 (Inception-ResNet-v2 and VGG-19) and CT, PET1 and PET3 (Resnet101). Finally, it can also be noticed that all network architectures underperformed in at least three different types of fused data, with the Inception-ResNet-v2 being the worst offender, scoring lower than 50% accuracies on 6 out of 10 groups of data.

Table 6.12: Feature level fusion classification accuracy (%) results. In bold are the best accuracies for each network architecture.

	Alexnet	Inception-ResNet-v2	VGG-16	Resnet101	VGG-19
PTV+PET1+PET2	42.86	50.00	42.86	57.14	50.00
PTV+PET1+PET3	50.00	50.00	50.00	50.00	35.71
PTV+PET2+PET3	**64.29**	42.86	42.86	42.86	35.71
PTV+CT+PET1	28.57	42.86	50.00	28.57	42.86
PTV+CT+PET2	50.00	57.14	**71.43**	35.71	57.14
PTV+CT+PET3	28.57	42.86	64.29	35.71	57.14
PET1+PET2+PET3	57.14	42.86	50.00	57.14	50.00
CT+PET1+PET2	50.00	35.71	50.00	50.00	35.71
CT+PET1+PET3	35.71	21.43	42.86	**64.29**	42.86
CT+PET2+PET3	28.57	**64.29**	50.00	57.14	**64.29**

6.3 Train from scratch

For this work, a convolutional neural network was also trained from scratch. It is composed of three convolutional layers, two max pooling layers, one fully connected layer and a binary output layer. Both single modality and feature-level fusion were applied in this section.

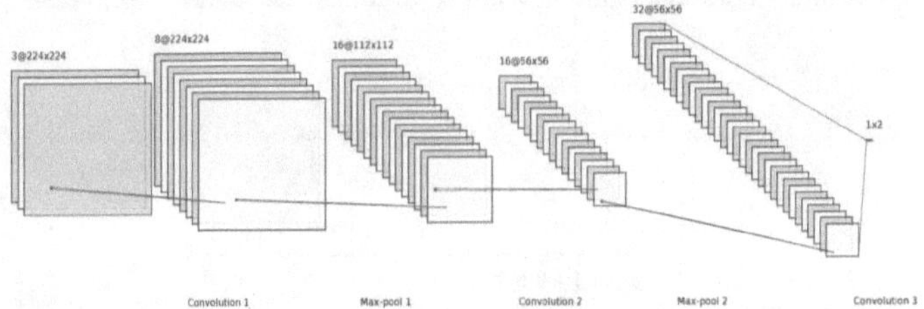

Figure 6.5: Architecture of the network trained from scratch

6.3.1 Single modality training

The results for the neural network trained from scratch are shown in Table 6.13. The network's results were lackluster in relation to previous sections, as the highest accuracy was 64.29% (PET2), while the remaining image modalities remained higher than or equal to 50%.

Table 6.13: Classification accuracy (%) for the used CNN. In bold are the best accuracies for each image type.

Image data	Train from scratch
PTV	50.00
CT	50.00
PET1	57.14
PET2	**64.29**
PET3	50.00

6.3.2 Feature level fusion

Finally, the feature level fusion results can be seen on Table 6.14. The best accuracy (64.29%) came from fusing the following sets of data:

- PTV+PET1+PET3

- PTV+CT+PET1

- CT+PET1+PET2

Moreover, the worst performances came from fusing all the PET data (PET1+PET2+PET3) and the CT images with the PET1 and PET3 data. Overall, there were not any improvements in comparison to single modality training from scratch, as the highest accuracies remained the same.

Table 6.14: Feature level fusion accuracies (%) for the network that was trained from scratch. In bold are the best accuracies.

Fusion data	Train from scratch
PTV+PET1+PET2	50.00
PTV+PET1+PET3	**64.29**
PTV+PET2+PET3	50.00
PTV+CT+PET1	**64.29**
PTV+CT+PET2	57.14
PTV+CT+PET3	57.14
PET1+PET2+PET3	42.86
CT+PET1+PET2	**64.29**
CT+PET1+PET3	42.86
CT+PET2+PET3	50.00

6.4 Conclusions

It can be seen that using pre-trained networks for feature extraction, while using "traditional classifiers" to separate between surgical and non-surgical candidates, is more effective than using transfer learning or training from scratch, which may be due to the small number of images used for training and testing. The best results for the deep learning pipeline can be seen on Table 6.15.

Table 6.15: Deep Learning selected results. In bold are the best accuracies.

Imaging	CNN	Classifier	Features	Accuracy (%)
PTV	VGG-16	Classification Trees	High-level	85.71
CT	VGG-16	Classification Ensembles	High-level	**100.00**
PET1	AlexNet	Support Vector Machines	Low-level	92.86
PET1	VGG-19	Discriminant Analysis	High-level	92.86
PET2	AlexNet	Classification Trees	Low-level	85.71
PET2	AlexNet	Classification Tree Ensembles	Low-level	85.71
PET2	VGG-16	Discriminant Analysis	Low-level	85.71
PET2	VGG-19	Discriminant Analysis	Low-level	85.71
PET3	ResNet-101	Classification Ensembles	High-level	92.86

The Confusion Matrix when extracting features from CT using VGG-16 and then classifying them with CE is given in Table 6.16.

Table 6.16: Confusion Matrix for the best deep learning model

	surgery not recommended	surgery recommended
does not need surgery	9	0
needs surgery	0	5

There is no observable trend in the image types, however, and single modality classification is also more effective than fusing different image modalities, while also being more computationally efficient.

Chapter 7.

Comparative Results

In this chapter, the best results from Chapter 5 and Chapter 6 were selected and not only compared with each other, but also with the results from the State of the Art Chapter, which are displayed in Table 7.1.

Table 7.1: State of the art results

Paper	Methods	Results	
		AUC	Accuracy
[70]	Logistic regression	0.71-0.79	-
[77]	SVM and Logistic Regression	-	57-100%
[35]	Evidential k-Nearest Neighborhood	-	100%
[36]	Evidential k-Nearest Neighborhood	0.77	89%
[6]	Logistic regression	0.58-0.78	-
[3]	3D-CNN	-	72-83%
[69]	3D-CNN	0.740	

Furthermore, in Table 7.2 the best results of the Traditional and Deep Learning methods are summarized. It can also be seen that these results go in line with the ones on the State of the Art chapter, with the VGG-16 high-level feature extraction method achieving 100% accuracy, with the CT data.

Table 7.2: Comparison between Traditional Learning (TL) and Deep Learning (DL) best results

Technique	Imaging	Method	Accuracy (%)
TL	PTV	Sequential Feature Selection; SVM	92.86
DL	CT	High-level VGG-16; Classification Ensembles	100.00

The ground is now laid to conduct a statistical test to evaluate the significance of the difference between the two methods. Two results are "significantly different" if the difference is statistically significant at the 1% level according to a paired two sided t-test, where each pair of data points consists of the estimates obtained by the two learning schemes being compared [9].

The statistical test did not reject the null hypothesis, at 1% significance level, that the pairwise difference between DL and TL results has a mean equal to zero. This was true both when comparing the final decisions and when comparing the predicted scores.

Chapter 8.

Conclusion and Future Work

According to the population-based Registo Oncológico Regional do Norte (RORENO), the Northern Portugal Cancer Registry, in 2013 around 211 new cases of esophageal cancer were diagnosed in the Northern Region, corresponding to an incidence rate of 7/10 [10]. This represents the highest incidence rate in the country, when compared to the Center, South and Azorean regions [55, 54]. The age-standardized incidence rate in men in the Northern Region of Portugal is also higher than the average observed for the European Region [24]. Until 2020 the number of incident cases of esophageal cancer in Northern Portugal is expected to increase more than 8%, to an estimated 227 new diagnoses [10].

Surgery remains the cornerstone of curative treatment in esophageal carcinoma patients with locoregional disease, despite the high surgical morbidity and the mortality rate due (50% and 5%, respectively) [30, 38]. Recent randomized trials have shown that neoadjuvant chemoradiotherapy significantly improved survival in patients with resectable tumours [30, 65, 60]. The complete pathological response in esophageal cancer, after neoadjuvant chemoradiotherapy, occurs in almost 50% of patients with squamous carcinomas and 23% of patients with adenocarcinomas [30]. However, and despite this high rate of complete pathological responses, these patients still undergo surgery due to the lack of sufficiently accurate mechanisms to determine the complete tumor response. Thus, the development of accurate diagnostic tools that could predict the complete pathological response is essential to avoid surgery, and the related morbi-mortality, in a significant percentage of patients.

The main goal of this work was to make a contribution in this field by comparing deep learning with traditional machine learning techniques. There is still a high prevalence of traditional techniques based on hand-crafted features in the field of Computer vision in esophageal cancer

[17]. Due to the unavailability of large datasets to train on and the multi-modality issue (i.e., need to incorporate information from different sources), deep learning methods are still in their infancy.

Data augmentation and transfer learning were applied in the deep learning method in order to compensate for the small number of data available. Moreover, several fusion techniques such as feature-level and decision-level fusion were also considered.

Even with the previously discussed challenges in deep learning, this method still managed to perfectly classify all examples, achieving 100% with the high-level CT image features, extracted using the VGG-16 network and classified using the Classification Ensembles model. Traditional learning achieved 92.86% accuracy only by using two shape features extracted from the PTV images, even though this method did not recommended surgery to a patient who should have undergone this procedure. A paired sample t-test was performed in these results, and it proved that the difference was not statistically significant.

This work represents some preliminary experiments and there are still some directions for the future. First and foremost, it would be of paramount importance to validate these results on larger datasets. Next, it would be interesting to experiment with 3D deep learning methods. Moreover, if 2D images are again considered, it would be interesting to develop a method to automatically select a slice from the volume (or a method to combine the results on several slices). For this, inspiration may be drawn from previous work on detection using deep learning or Bayesian surprise [14, 16]. Data fusion at input level for deep learning (for instance, inserting a different image type in each channel) will also be explored [15]. Data augmentation with anatomic considerations [15] and oversampling [18, 39] might help overcoming the data imbalance problem (64% of the patients in the dataset had a complete pathological response, while 36% had an incomplete response). For being a medical application, we are also aware of the importance of interpretability [2].

In summary, various machine learning techniques in a biomedical context were explored, with the aim of advancing the state of the art in the field of computer vision in esophageal cancer. However, it is foreseen that the observation here made may be also applicable to other fields that also face the same difficulties, such as multi-modality and few labelled data.

Appendices

Chapter A.
Network Architectures

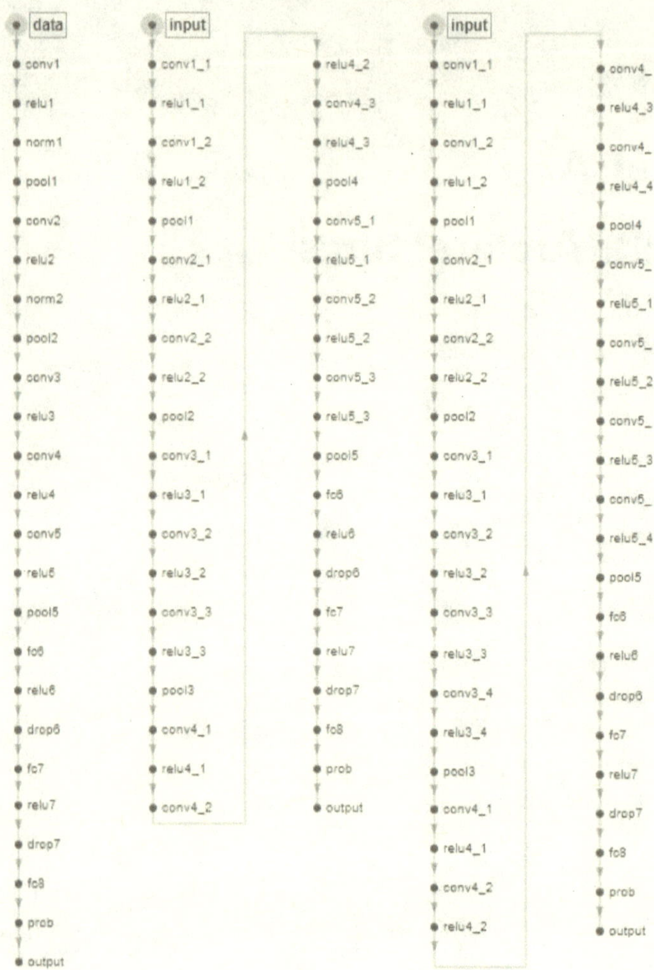

Figure A.1: AlexNet, VGG-16 and VGG-19 (left to right) network architectures used for transfer learning and deep learning feature extraction.

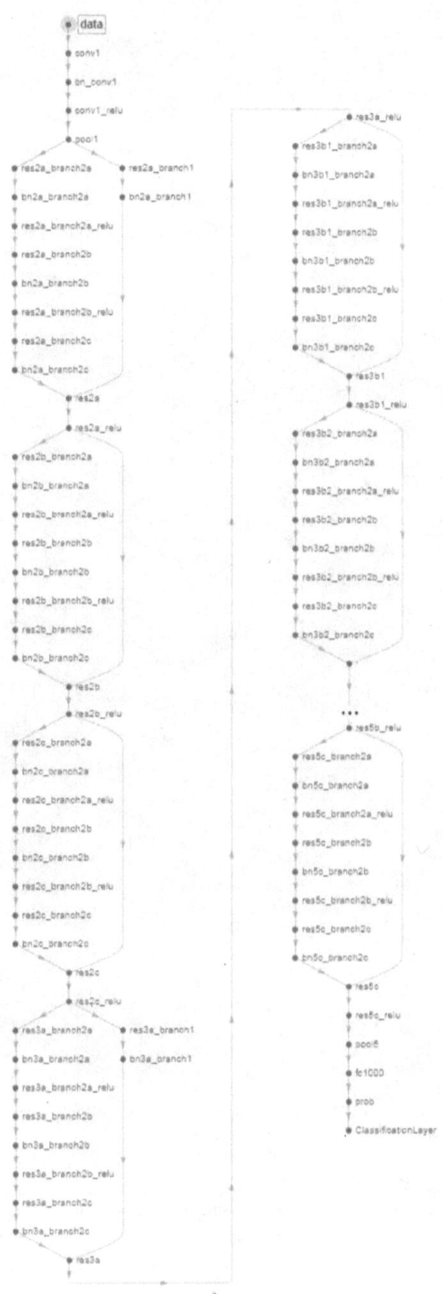

Figure A.2: ResNet-101 network architecture used for transfer learning and deep learning feature extraction. Due to the complexity of the architecture, only a partial illustration was performed.

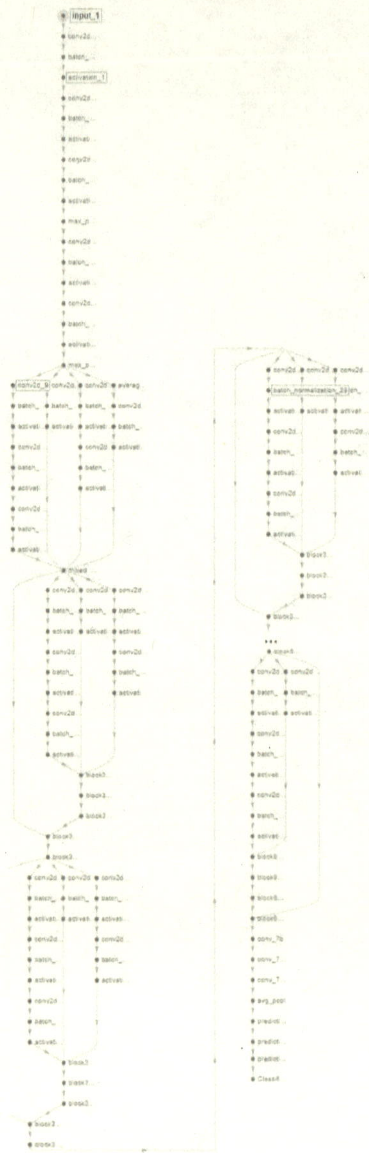

Figure A.3: InceptionResNetv2 network architecture used for transfer learning and deep learning feature extraction. Due to the complexity of the architecture, only a partial illustration was performed.

Chapter B.
RECPAD Poster and Article

Classifying very small multi-modal data: application oesophagic early-stage cancers

Jorge Ferreira[1], Inês Domingues[2], João Santos[2]

1 Faculty of Sciences of University of Porto
2 IPO Porto Research Centre (CI-IPOP), Radiobiology and Radiation Protection Group, Medical Physics

Abstract

Esophageal cancer is a disease with a high prevalence which can be evaluated by a variety of imaging modalities, including: Endoscopy, CT and PET. In some cases, however, it is known that surgery could be avoided. Computer vision techniques could provide a valuable help in the analysis of these images, for it would allow an enhancement in diagnostic and staging accuracies, a decrease in medical workflow time and preventing patients' loss of quality of life.

Introduction

Esophageal cancer (EC) is one of the most reported malignancies, ranking seventh in terms of incidence (572,000 new cases) and sixth in general mortality (509,000 deaths). It also can be evaluated by a variety of imaging modalities, as shown in Figure 1: Endoscopy, Computed Tomography (CT) and Positron Emition Tomography (PET).

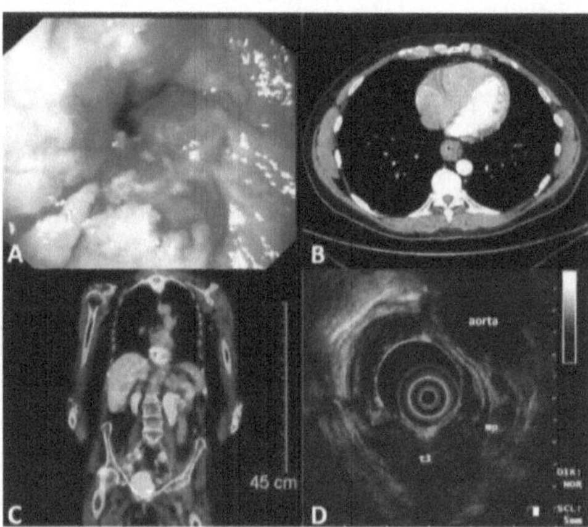

Figure 1:Esophageal cancer staging (adapted from [2]): (A) Advanced lower esophageal adenocarcinoma diagnosed at endoscopy; (B) Subsequent CT; (C) PET-CT imaging; (D) Endoscopic ultrasound.

Objective

The goal of this work is to showcase the applications of deep learning and computer vision in an under-explored context, the domain of esophageal cancer, as well as new ways to deal with small and multi-modal data.

Methodology

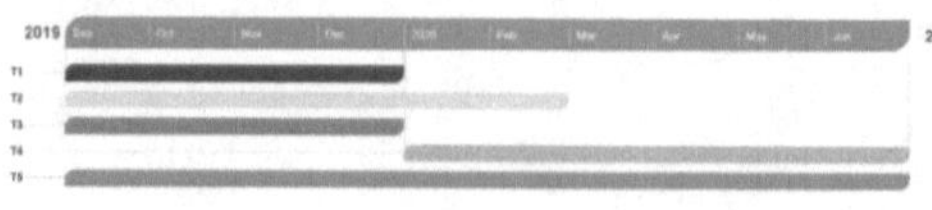

Figure 2:Planning roadmap

The Planning Roadmap of the present research project in Figure 2 includes the following tasks:

- T1: Background knowledge in deep learning techniques in computer vision, as well as the study of the characteristics of EC.
- T2: Search and analysis of public and private databases.
- T3: Literature review based on the paper [1].
- T4: Test, evaluation and comparison among State of the art techniques.
- T5: Dissemination of the work through a Master's thesis and presentation, as well as a journal paper.

Conclusion

The present work aims at exploring various deep learning techniques in a biomedical context and thus advancing the state of the art in the field of computer vision in esophageal cancer. However, we do foresee that some of the contributions may be also applicable to other fields that also face the same difficulties, such as multi-modality and few labelled data.

References

[1] I. Domingues, I. L. Sampaio, H. Duarte, J. A. M. dos Santos, and P. H. Abreu. Computer vision in esophageal cancer: a literature review. *IEEE Access*, 7(1):103080–103094, 2019. doi: 10.1109/ACCESS.2019.2930891.

[2] A. D. Hopper and J. A. Campbell. Early diagnosis of oesophageal cancer improves outcomes. *Practitioner*, 260(1791):23–28, 2016.

Acknowledgements

This article is a result of the project NORTE-01-0145-FEDER-000027, supported by Norte Portugal Regional Operational Programme (NORTE 2020), under the PORTUGAL 2020 Partnership Agreement, through the European Regional Development Fund (ERDF).

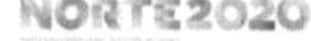
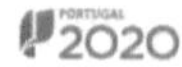
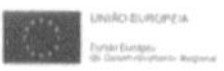

Jorge Filipe Santos Ferreira[1]
up201306524@fc.up.pt

Inês Domingues[2]
inesdomingues@gmail.com

João Santos[2]
joao.santos@ipoporto.min-saude.pt

[1] Faculdade de Ciências
Universidade do Porto
Portugal

[2] Medical Physics
Radiobiology and Radiation Protection Group
IPO Porto Research Centre (CI-IPOP)

Abstract

Esophageal cancer is a disease with a high prevalence which can be evaluated by a variety of imaging modalities, including Endoscopy, CT, and PET. Computer vision techniques could provide a valuable help in the analysis of these images decreasing the medical workflow time and enhancing diagnostic and staging accuracy.

Current guidelines for esophageal treatment typically include neoadjuvant radiochemotherapy followed by surgery. In some cases, however, it is known from post-surgery anatomopathologic data, that surgery could be avoided. Computer vision could present solutions aiming at finding criteria for the clear separation between surgical and non-surgical candidates, avoiding the loss of quality of life and surgery associated comorbilities.

The development of these techniques on the present application encompasses two main difficulties. One is the multi-modality of the data. We want to leverage not only on the different types of images previously mentioned, but also on non-image data such as medical reports and clinical data. The other main difficulty is the existence of small training data. Data augmentation and transfer learning present some possible solutions to this problem.

1 Introduction

Esophageal Cancer (EC) is, globally, one of the most frequently reported malignancies [3, 6]. This disease ranks seventh in terms of incidence (572,000 new cases) and sixth in general mortality (509,000 deaths), the latter meaning that esophageal cancer will account for an estimated one in every 20 deaths from cancer in 2018 [2].

As with other diseases of the upper GastroIntestinal (GI) tract, EC can be evaluated by a variety of imaging modalities [1, 4], including (Figure 1):

- Endoscopy

    - Application: endoscopy with biopsy is used to diagnose EC.

    - Main advantages: permits direct inspection and biopsy of the esophageal mucosa for histologic diagnosis.

    - Main disadvantages: it is an invasive technique and operator dependent.

- Computed Tomography (CT)

    - Application: useful in distinguishing between patients with early cancer who need further evaluation with Endoscopy and those were the tumour is already invading other structures; used for tumour delineation during radiotherapy planning.

    - Main advantages: reliable in determining resectability.

    - Main disadvantages: CT is unable to distinguish the wall layers of the oesophagus to determine the depth of tumour infiltration.

- Positron Emission Tomography (PET)

    - Application: Fluorodesoxiglicose (FDG)-PET is a established imaging technique for staging EC, being the most important role of this modality the detection of distant metastases.

    - Main advantages: assessing of metabolic function, high sensibility, high reproducibility (when complying with the acquisition standards), and existence of quantitative measurements such as SUV (Standardized Uptake Value).

    - Main disadvantages: low spatial resolution when compared with other imaging techniques, low specificity of 18F-FDG-PET, and still a lack of commercial availability of other pharmaceuticals beyond F-18:FDG.

A summary of the different imaging techniques in EC used in clinical practice for diagnosis, TNM-staging, tumour delineation for Radiotherapy (RT), and treatment response assessment, is given in Table 1.

Table 1: Imaging techniques in esophageal cancer used for diagnosis, TNM-staging, tumour delineation for RT, and treatment response assessment [1]

	Endoscopy	CT	PET
Diagnosis	✓		
T-Staging	✓	✓	
N-Staging	✓	✓	✓
M-Staging		✓	✓
Tumour delineation for RT		✓	✓
Evaluation of response	✓	✓	✓

As observed in [1], there is still a high prevalence of traditional techniques based on hand-crafted features in the field of Computer vision in esophageal cancer, while deep learning is still in the early stages of adoption. This may due to two main difficulties, the need to incorporate information from different sources (multi-modality) and the unavailability of large datasets to train the models on. The main goal of this work is thus to develop methods that can return useful models in this challenging setting.

2 Methodology

The Planning Roadmap of the present research project is shown in Figure 2 and includes the following tasks:

- T1: Familiarisation with the problem

- T2: Database collection

- T3: Literature review

- T4: Implementation of techniques for identification of patients that do not need surgery

- T5: Dissemination of the work

In T1, the characteristics of the esophageal cancer will be studied, given particular attention to the differences between surgical and non-surgical candidates and how these aspects manifest in the different imaging modalities, namely Endoscopy, CT and PET. Background knowledge on deep learning techniques in the field of computer vision will also be built. Here, particular attention will be given to methods that incorporate different sources of images and that can cope with few labelled data. It is important to mention that we are interested not only in the setting when all the image types are present for every example, but also in methods that can deal with missing information for one or more modalities in one or

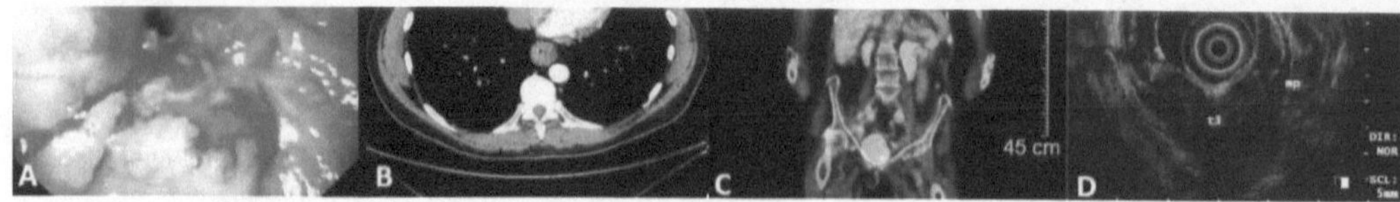

Figure 1: Esophageal cancer staging (adapted from [5]): (A) Advanced lower esophageal adenocarcinoma diagnosed at endoscopy; (B) Subsequent CT; (C) PET-CT imaging; (D) Endoscopic ultrasound.

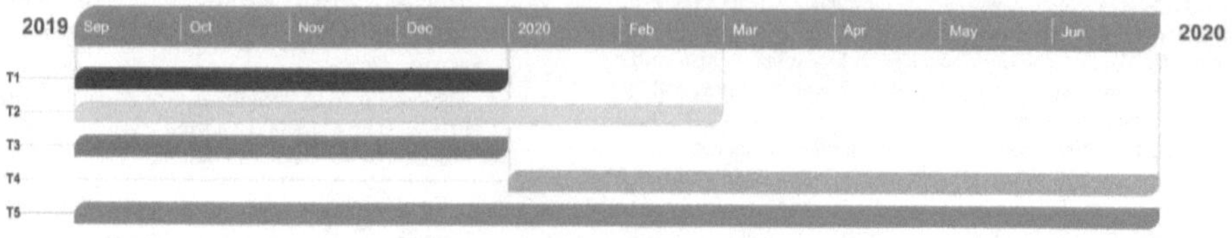

Figure 2: Planning Roadmap.

more instances, since some patients may not have gone through all imaging exams. Medical doctors need to decide if the benefits of performing an exam outweigh the harms such as the radiation applied to the patient and also the costs in time and money. Moreover, some exams may not be possible to perform in some patients. To cope with few labelled data, we foresee the use of publicity available datasets, the application of transfer learning techniques, and also the use of semi supervised methods (since unlabelled data is easier to obtain the medical field).

The second task, T2, will consist in both the search for publicly available databases, and also the collection of a private database from IPO-Porto. A list of publicly available datasets can be found in [1], which includes MICCAI 2015 "EndoVis", ISBI 2016 "AIDA-E", esophageal IPCL, ISBI 2019 "EAD", and "GastroAtlas" for Endoscopy; and MIC-CAI 2015 and TCGA-ESCA for CT. It is clear that endoscopy is the modality that has raised most interest in the community, followed by CT, while there are no publicly available databases for PET. This list will be updated to include more datasets, in case any has been more recently made available. The private database will be built respecting the privacy of the patient and thus all personal information will be anonymized.

A literature review on Computer vision in esophageal cancer will be performed in T3. This will have as basis the paper [1], that will be updated and complement if necessary. Again, special attention will be given on how multimodality and the existence of few labelled data have been explored in the context of esophageal cancer.

The main part of this work is concentrated on task T4, where the development is performed. State of the art techniques will be tested and evaluated with the collected dataset composed of both public and private images. Whenever possible, implementations made available by the original authors will be used. We do foresee, however, that besides the comparison of existing techniques, new scientific contributions will come from this work, built upon all the gathered knowledge and applied in this still under-explored context of the use of deep learning for the management of esophageal cancer.

Finally, task T5 focus on the dissemination of the work. This conference paper represents a first component of this task. A Master book report and presentation will also result from this project. Moreover, new scientific contributions will be published in the form of a journal paper. If the ethics committee of IPO authorises, the collected and anonymous database will also be made available.

3 Conclusions

The present work aims at exploring various deep learning techniques in a biomedical context and thus advancing the state of the art in the field of computer vision in esophageal cancer. However, we do foresee that some of the contributions may be also applicable to other fields that also face the same difficulties, such as multi-modality and few labelled data.

4 Acknowledgements

This article is a result of the project NORTE-01-0145-FEDER-000027, supported by Norte Portugal Regional Operational Programme (NORTE 2020), under the PORTUGAL 2020 Partnership Agreement, through the European Regional Development Fund (ERDF).

References

[1] Inês Domingues, Inês Lucena Sampaio, Hugo Duarte, João António Miranda dos Santos, and Pedro Henriques Abreu. Computer vision in esophageal cancer: a literature review. *IEEE Access*, 7(1): 103080–103094, 2019. doi: 10.1109/ACCESS.2019.2930891.

[2] F. Bray, Jacques Ferlay, Isabelle Soerjomataram, Rebecca L. Siegel;, Lindsey A. Torre;, and Ahmedin Jemal. Global Cancer Statistics 2018: GLOBOCAN Estimates of Incidence and Mortality Worldwide for 36 Cancers in 185 Countries. *CA: A Cancer Journal for Clinicians*, 2018. ISSN 00079235. doi: 10.3322/caac.21492.

[3] J Ferlay, I Soerjomataram, and M Ervik. GLOBOCAN 2012v1.0, Cancer Incidence and Mortality Worldwide, 2013.

[4] Kieran Foley, John Findlay, and Vicky Goh. Novel imaging techniques in staging oesophageal cancer. *Best Practice and Research in Clinical Gastroenterology*, 2018. ISSN 15216918. doi: S1521691818300921.

[5] Andrew D Hopper and Jennifer A Campbell. Early diagnosis of oesophageal cancer improves outcomes. *Practitioner*, 260(1791):23–28, 2016.

[6] Martin C S Wong, Willie Hamilton, David C Whiteman, Johnny Y Jiang, Youlin Qiao, Franklin D H Fung, Harry H X Wang, Philip W Y Chiu, Enders K W Ng, Justin C Y Wu, Jun Yu, Francis K L Chan, and Joseph J Y Sung. Global Incidence and mortality of oesophageal cancer and their correlation with socioeconomic indicators temporal patterns and trends in 41 countries. *Scientific Reports*, 8(1):1–13, 2018. ISSN 20452322. doi: 10.1038/s41598-018-19819-8.

Chapter C.
Scientific Paper

Classification of oesophagic early-stage cancers: deep learning versus traditional learning approaches

Jorge Ferreira
Faculdade de Ciências da Universidade do Porto (FCUP)
Porto, Portugal
up201306524@fc.up.pt

Inês Domingues
Medical Physics, Radiobiology and Radiation Protection Group
IPO Porto Research Centre (CI-IPOP)
inesdomingues@gmail.com

Olga Sousa
Radioncology Department
Portuguese Institute of Oncology of Porto (IPO-Porto)
Porto, Portugal

Inês Lucena Sampaio
Medical Physics, Radiobiology and Radiation Protection Group,
IPO Porto Research Centre (CI-IPOP)
Nuclear Medicine Department, IPO-Porto

João A. M. Santos
Medical Physics Department, Portuguese Institute of Oncology of Porto (IPO-Porto)
Instituto de Ciências Biomédicas Abel Salazar da Universidade do Porto
Porto, Portugal
joao.santos@ipoporto.min-saude.pt

Abstract—Esophageal cancer is a disease with a high prevalence which can be evaluated by a variety of imaging modalities. Computer vision techniques could provide a valuable help in the analysis of these images, for it would allow an enhancement in diagnostic and staging accuracies, a decrease in medical workflow time and preventing patients' loss of quality of life.

Traditional learning techniques are frequently used in the biomedical imaging field, and deep learning algorithms are starting to see their rise in usage in this field as well. In this paper, both traditional and deep learning algorithms are applied on a dataset provided by Instituto Português de Oncologia (IPO) consisting of CT and three PET scans acquired at different treatment phases of 14 patients with oesophageal cancer.

The main goal is to distinguish patients that need surgery from the ones that do not. To achieve this goal, we have framed this question as a two-class classification problem. The traditional learning method consisted of manually extracting the features and apply feature selection algorithms for further classification. Feature level and decision level fusion were also conducted. The deep learning method consisted of using convolutional neural networks (both pretrained and trained from scratch) to extract and classify the image features on 2D images composed of 3 slices for all the data used in this work. Moreover, traditional and deep learning techniques were used simultaneously, where the features were extracted and selected by a pretrained network and classified using the traditional learning classifiers.

Traditional Learning methods achieved 92.86% accuracy, while for feature extraction with deep learning followed by classification with a traditional classifier was able to reach 100% accuracy. The difference has, however, proven not to be statistically significant. In this way, for this particular problem and conditions, it can be said that traditional techniques are capable of achieving results as good as with deep learning.

Index Terms—Oesophagic cancer, PET, CT, Classification, Deep Learning, Traditional Learning

I. Introduction

Esophageal Cancer (EC) is, globally, one of the most frequently reported malignancies [12], [19]. This disease ranks seventh in terms of incidence (572,000 new cases) and sixth in general mortality (509,000 deaths), the latter meaning that EC will account for an estimated one in every 20 deaths from cancer in 2018 [4].

As with other diseases of the upper Gastrointestinal (GI) tract, EC can be evaluated by a variety of imaging modalities [11], [14], including CT and PET. Computer vision techniques could provide a valuable help in the analysis of these images decreasing the medical workflow time and enhancing diagnostic and staging accuracy.

Current guidelines for esophageal treatment typically include neoadjuvant radiochemotherapy followed by surgery. In some cases, however, it is known from postsurgery anatomopathologic data, that surgery could be avoided. Computer vision could present solutions aiming at finding criteria for the clear separation between surgical and non-surgical candidates, avoiding the loss of quality of life and surgery associated comorbilities.

The development of these techniques on the present application encompasses two main difficulties. One is the multimodality of the data. We want to leverage all of the different types of images available, such as PET and CT. The other main difficulty is the existence of small training data. Data

This work is financed by National Funds through the Portuguese funding agency, FCT - Fundação para a Ciência Tecnologia within project UIDP/00776/2020 and the project NORTE-01-0145-FEDER-000027, supported by Norte Portugal Regional Operational Programme (NORTE 2020), under the PORTUGAL 2020 Partnership Agreement, through the European Regional Development Fund (ERDF).

augmentation and transfer learning present some possible solutions to this problem.

The present document shows experiments on the classification of PET and CT scans of patients with esophageal cancer into two classes, patients that need surgery and patients that do not need surgery. The contributions include:

- Presentation of a new database of patients with oesophagic early-stage cancer, with CT and three PET scans (acquired at different treatment phases) for each patient
- A formalisation of the problem as identification of patients that do not need surgery
- Radiomic and automatic features extracted from both PET and CT
- Traditional learning including fusion at both feature and decision level, feature selection, and several state of the art classifiers
- Different uses of deep learning, as feature extractor, using pre-trained classification networks, and an architecture that was trained from scratch
- Formal evaluation and comparison (both among the best tested methods and with the state of the art works) with significance proved by statistical tests

The remaining of this document is organised as follows. In Section II an overview of previous work done in related fields is done. The database used for the experiments is described in Section III. Section IV presents and illustrated the machine learning pipelines, both under the traditional philosophy and at the light of deep learning. Results are presented in Section V and the document finishes in Section VI with some conclusions and directions to future work.

II. STATE OF THE ART

A comprehensive analysis of the literature was performed on [11]. It can be noticed that there is no other work that explicitly focus on identifying patients that do not need surgery. There are, however, some works that are close to the present work in the sense that deal with binary classification problems. Table I explores these works by presenting the main methods used and results achieved.

TABLE I
STATE OF THE ART

Paper	Methods	Results	
		AUC	Accuracy
[21]	Logistic regression	0.71-0.79	-
[22]	SVM and Logistic Regression	-	57-100%
[16]	Evidential k-Nearest Neighborhood	-	100%
[15]	Evidential k-Nearest Neighborhood	0.77	89%
[3]	Logistic regression	0.58-0.78	-
[2]	3D-CNN	-	72-83%
[20]	3D-CNN	0.740	

It should be noted that, across all the works on Table I, only [3] combined information from both CT and PET. Moreover, no temporal information is used. In the present work, we combine information from CT and three PET scans performed at different treatment phases.

III. DATASET

A prospective cohort study of consecutively sampled patients allocated to neoadjuvant chemo-radiotherapy (NCRT) regimen according to local protocols was performed. For this particular early stage, curative, resectable disease cohort of patients, the inclusion criteria was diagnosis of squamous cell carcinoma, undifferentiated carcinoma or adenocarcinoma of esophageal or esophagealgastric junction (Siewert I e II) and clinical Stage II or III disease, according to American Joint Committee on Cancer Staging classification, 7th edition. All patients presented the upper border of the tumour at least 3 cm below the upper esophageal sphincter. All patient signed an informed consent and the study was approved by the institution ethics committee. Exclusion criteria included pregnant or lactating women, previous thoracic radiotherapy, Impaired haematological, hepatic, renal or pulmonary function defined, neutrophils count $< 1.5 \times 10^9$/L, platelet count $< 100 \times 10^9$/L, serum concentration of total bilirubin > 1.5 x ULN (upper limit of normal range), creatinine > 120 mcmol/L, FEV1 (Forced expiratory volume in 1 second) < 1.5 L and active infection or other medical condition that prevents the patient from receiving the planed treatment.

Molecular imaging (PET/CT) images were acquired at three time points (see Figure):

- Baseline study: 18-Fluoro (18-F)-FDG PET/CT performed with a maximum interval of 21 days until the start of CRT; These studies will be denominated PET1.
- Early molecular imaging study: 18-F-FDG PET/CT, performed preferably on the 8th after the start of CRT (before the 2nd chemotherapy cycle); These studies will be denominated PET2.
- Post CRT study: 18-F-FDG PET/CT, performed 6 weeks after CRT; These studies will be denominated PET3.

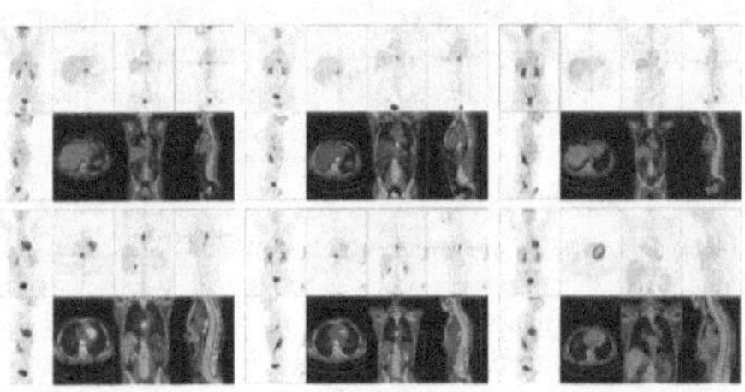

Fig. 1. Examples of scans from the database. Top: patient with complete pathological response; Bottom: patient with incomplete pathological response;. Left: Baseline, Middle: Early molecular imaging, Right: Post Chemoradiotherapy.

Delineation of regions of interest (including the PTV - planning treatment volume), made on the baseline CT are also available.

The dataset is composed of 14 patients and 3 PET images for each one, totalling 42 images, where 9 patients had a complete pathological response and 5 had an incomplete response.

Pre-processing: All scans were resampled to a voxel size of 4x4x4. PET scans were rotated to be in the same orientation as CT scans. For co-registration, the technique proposed in [18] was used.

IV. METHODS

In this section we detail the techniques implemented, in particular the ones based on traditional learning and then the ones based on deep learning [10].

A. Traditional Learning

The full pipeline of the Traditional Learning approach is presented in Figure 2.

Traditional learning was performed recurring to hand-crafted features. Shape and intensity features were extracted. Shape features were extracted from the PTV and include characteristics such as the centroid, convex volume, extend, solidity, surface area, volume, and other typically used features. Intensity features were extracted for CT and each one of the three PETs, within the region defined by the PTV, and include maximum, average, and minimum intensities, standard deviation of the intensities, and the weighted centroid.

A total of 42 features were extracted, 22 shape features for the PTV plus 5 intensity features for each of the 4 scans (CT, first PET, second PET and third PET).

Tested classifiers include Classification Trees (CT), Discriminant Analysis (DA), k-Nearest Neighbours (kNN), Naive Bayes (NB), Support Vector Machines (SVM), Classification Tree Ensembles (CTE) and Classification Ensembles (CE).

Fusion was performed at feature level (where features are concatenated), and at decision level (both by majority voting and by averaging the results of the individual classifiers). For the feature level fusion, all combinations of the 5 sets of features with the 7 classifiers were tested.

Finally, some feature selection algorithms were attempted: Minimum Redundancy Maximum Relevance (MRMR), neighborhood component analysis (NCA), Laplacian Score, ReliefF algorithm, and Sequential feature selection.

B. Deep Learning

Deep learning techniques in two-dimensions were attempted. For that, the slice with the biggest PTV area was first identified. Then, that slice, the previous one and the one after were retrieved to form 2D images with 3 channels. Examples retrieved from two patients are given in Figure 3.

As we are dealing with a small dataset [13], transfer learning approaches were favoured.

Pre-trained CNNs (Alexnet, Resnet-101, VGG-16, Inception-ResNet-v2 and VGG-19) were first used as feature extractors (this will be referred to as the first strategy). Convolutional Neural Networks perform a hierarchical construction of an input image: earlier layers process the low-level features from the input images, and deeper layers build more complex structures (i.e., high-level features) based on the low-level features. Both low-level and high-level features were extracted from the Pre-trained CNNs and were classified using the same traditional classifiers as above (Figure 4).

The pipeline is given in Figure 5. For this method, all images were resized to $224 \times 224 \times 3$ and data augmentation was performed on the training images: the images were rotated 45 degrees, both anticlockwise and clockwise, reflections (in the x axis) and translations of 30 pixels were also applied; moreover, the data also suffered scaling operations, to 90% and 110% of their original size.

A different technique was to use the above mentioned models and adjust the final layers so they could perform the desired classification task (this will be referred to as the second strategy), Figure 6. In this way, the last learnable layer of each network was replaced by a fully connected layer with two outputs representing the two classes of interest (needs surgery and does not need surgery). Resizing and data augmentation was performed as above. Training was endured with Adam optimizer, using a batch size of one, six maximum epochs, and an initial learning rate of 3×10^{-4}.

For comparison purposes, a new network, to be trained from scratch was also designed (this will be referred to as the third strategy). Due to the small size of the dataset, the network was kept small with three convolutional layers, two max pooling layers, three ReLU layers, one fully connected layer, a softmax layer and a binary output layer. A diagram of this network is given in Figure 7. Resizing and data augmentation was performed as above. Training was endured with Adam optimiser, using a batch size of one, six maximum epochs, and an initial learning rate of 0.01.

V. RESULTS

This section is organised into several parts. First, a description of the evaluation methodology is given. Next results are presented for the traditional techniques. The next parts present results for the deep learning methods. Finally, a comparison between the best model of each philosophy is given.

A. Evaluation methodology

Leave-one-patient-out cross validation was used for evaluation. Accuracy and Confusion matrices were chosen to quantify the results.

B. Traditional Learning

The set of experiments is of the order of 2×10^3 (31 combinations of features, 6 feature selection techniques, 6 classifiers, and 2 decision fusion methods). For the sake of brevity, only selected results are presented in Table II.

It can be seen from the table, that PTV seems to convey important information to discriminate patients that need surgery from the ones that do not. Moreover, feature selection, and fusion (both at feature and at decision levels) do not seem to be able to improve these results. Although not improving the final accuracy, the classifier with only two features chosen by Sequential feature selection, was able to achieve the same results as the classifier with the full set of features.

For this particular problem, it would be worse to not perform a surgery in a patient that needed it than to perform a surgery in

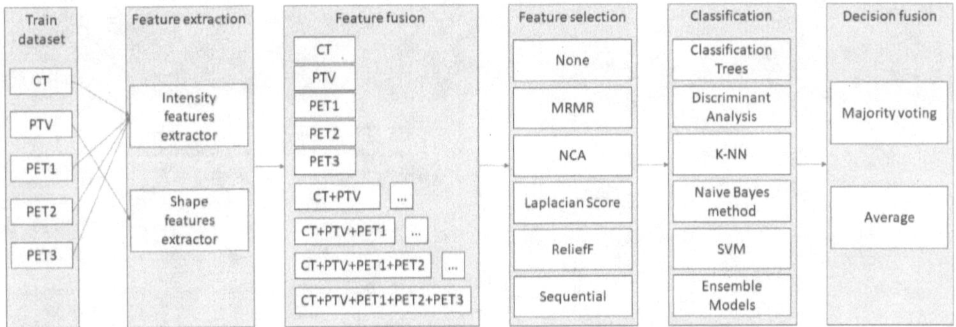

Fig. 2. Traditional Learning pipeline

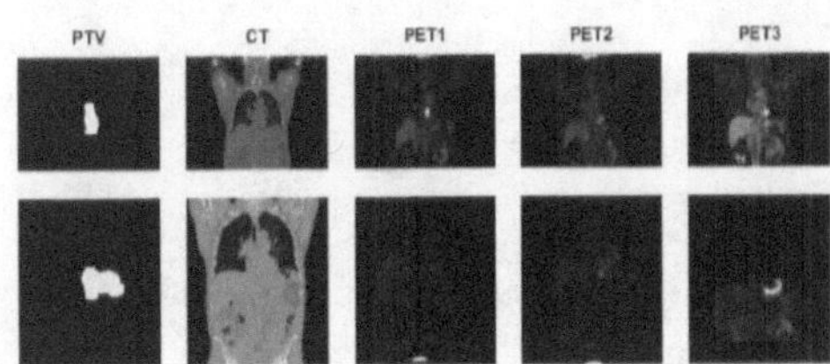

Fig. 3. Selected slices from two patients.

TABLE II
TRADITIONAL LEARNING SELECTED RESULTS

Imaging	Feature selection	Classifier	Accuracy (%)
PTV	none	DA	92.86
CT	none	SVM	71.43
CT	none	CTE	71.43
PET1	none	kNN	64.29
PET1	none	NB	64.29
PET2	none	kNN	64.29
PET2	none	NB	64.29
PET3	none	kNN	64.29
PET3	none	NB	64.29
PTV	Sequential	SVM	92.86

patients that do not need it (which is what is made in practice nowadays). In this way, it is important to access not only the overall accuracy, but also the type of errors that are made. The confusion matrix of the best model (SVM trained with the two chosen features extracted from the PTV) is given in Table III. It can be seen that one patient that need surgery would be recommended not to have surgery.

TABLE III
CONFUSION MATRIX FOR THE BEST TRADITIONAL MODEL

	surgery not recommended	surgery recommended
does not need surgery	64%	0%
needs surgery	7%	29%

Illustrative results of correctly and incorrectly classified cases are given in Figure 8. It is clear the similarity between the PTV of the two cases that were recommended by the SVM not to perform surgery, although the patient on the left did not needed surgery, but the patient on the middle did needed it and was thus incorrectly classified.

C. Deep Learning

A total of 380 experiments have been performed (5 types of images, 3 strategies, 5 deep architectures for the first two strategies, 7 traditional classifiers for the first strategy, and 2 types of features for the first strategy). For the sake of brevity, only selected results are presented in Table IV.

TABLE IV
DEEP LEARNING SELECTED RESULTS (STRATEGY 1).

Imaging	CNN	Classifier	Features	Accuracy (%)
PTV	VGG-16	CT	High-level	85.71
CT	VGG-16	CE	High-level	100.00
PET1	AlexNet	SVM	Low-level	92.86
PET1	VGG-19	DA	High-level	92.86
PET2	AlexNet	CT	Low-level	85.71
PET2	AlexNet	CTE	Low-level	85.71
PET2	VGG-16	DA	Low-level	85.71
PET2	VGG-19	DA	Low-level	85.71
PET3	ResNet-101	CE	High-level	92.86

Here, the first strategy (to use pre-trained networks as feature extractors) outperformed all the others. This may be due to the small size of the dataset. Concerning the type of features, no clear trend is observed. A possible direction for future work is to experiment concatenating high and low level features.

The Confusion Matrix when extracting features from CT using VGG-16 and then classifying them with CE is given in Table V.

D. Comparison

A summary of the best results achieved with each technique is displayed in Table VI. When relating these results with the

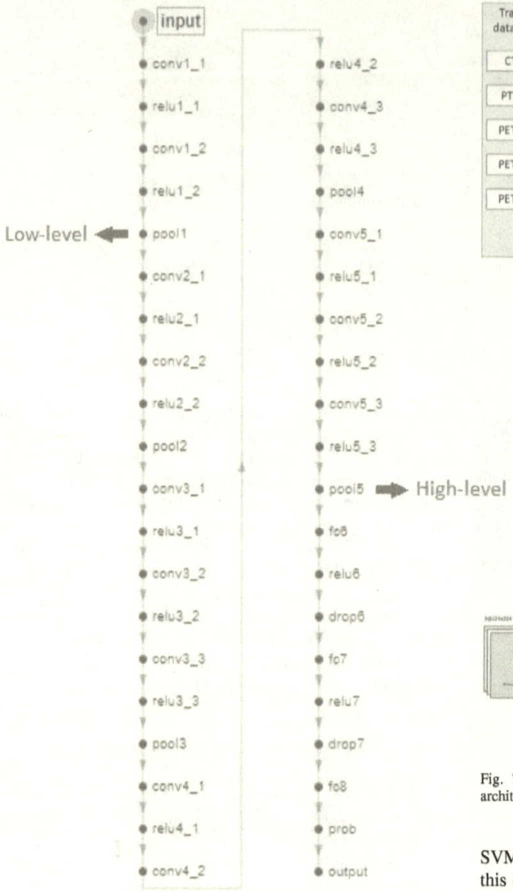

input

Low-level ← pool1

conv1_1 · relu1_1 · conv1_2 · relu1_2 · pool1 · conv2_1 · relu2_1 · conv2_2 · relu2_2 · pool2 · conv3_1 · relu3_1 · conv3_2 · relu3_2 · conv3_3 · relu3_3 · pool3 · conv4_1 · relu4_1 · conv4_2

relu4_2 · conv4_3 · relu4_3 · pool4 · conv5_1 · relu5_1 · conv5_2 · relu5_2 · conv5_3 · relu5_3 · pool5 → High-level · fc6 · relu6 · drop6 · fc7 · relu7 · drop7 · fc8 · prob · output

Fig. 4. Illustration of High and Low level features on VGG-16 network.

TABLE V

CONFUSION MATRIX FOR THE BEST DEEP LEARNING MODEL

	surgery not recommended	surgery recommended
does not need surgery	64%	0%
needs surgery	0%	36%

Train dataset	Feature extraction	Feature selection	Classification
CT	AlexNet		Classification Trees
PTV	Resnet-101		Discriminant Analysis
PET1	VGG-16	Low-level	K-NN
PET2	Inception-ResNet-v2	High-level	Naive Bayes method
PET3	VGG-19		SVM
			Ensemble Models

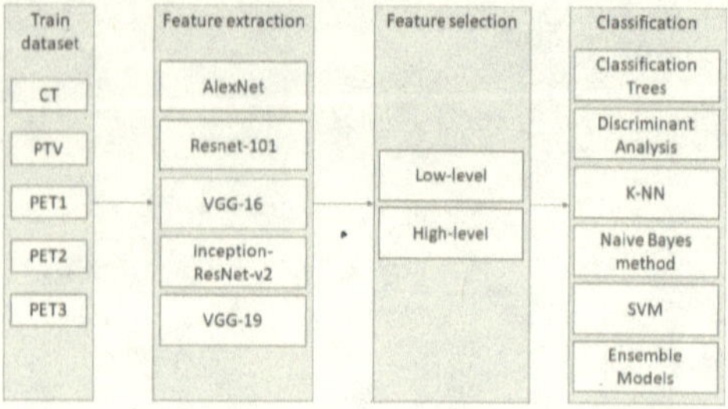

Fig. 5. Deep Learning for feature extraction (transfer learning).

Train dataset	Classification
CT	AlexNet
PTV	Resnet-101
PET1	VGG-16
PET2	Inception-ResNet-v2
PET3	VGG-19

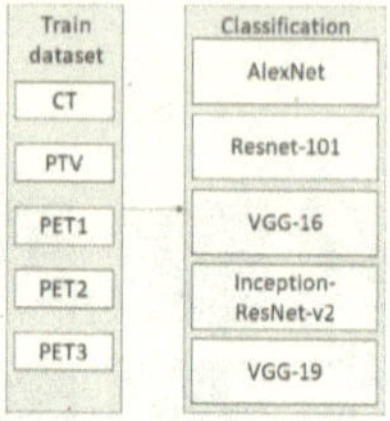

Fig. 6. Deep Learning for classification (transfer learning).

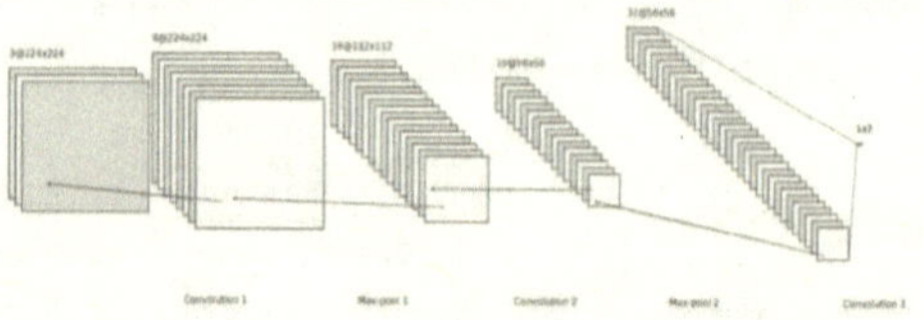

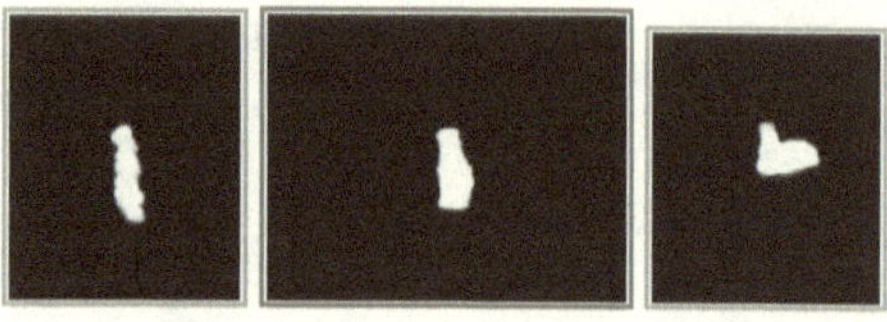

Fig. 7. Deep Learning for classification (trained from scratch network architecture).

SVM), it is important to evaluate the statistical significance of this difference.

Throughout this section we speak of two results as being "significantly different" if the difference is statistically significant at the 1% level according to a paired two sided t-test, where each pair of data points consists of the estimates

ones achieved in the state of the art (Table I), we see similar performances with accuracy values reaching 100%.

Although Deep Learning with CT high level features extracted from VGG-16 and then classified with CE seem to outperform the best traditional method (two PTV features chosen by Sequential Feature Selection and then classified using

Fig. 8. Best traditional model results (only the slice with the biggest PTV area is shown). Left: Correctly classified patient that does not need surgery; Middle: Incorrectly classified patient that needs surgery; Right: Correctly classified patient that needs surgery.

TABLE VI

COMPARISON BETWEEN TRADITIONAL LEARNING (TL) AND DEEP
LEARNING (DL) BEST RESULTS

Technique	Imaging	Method	Accuracy (%)
TL	PTV	Sequential Feature Selection; SVM	92.86
DL	CT	High-level VGG-16; CE	100.00

obtained by the two learning schemes being compared [5].

The statistical test did not reject the null hypothesis, at 1% significance level, that the pairwise difference between DL and TL results has a mean equal to zero. This was true both when comparing the final decisions and when comparing the predicted scores.

VI. CONCLUSIONS

As observed in [11], there is still a high prevalence of traditional techniques based on hand-crafted features in the field of Computer vision in esophageal cancer, while deep learning is in the early stages of adoption. This may due to two main difficulties, the need to incorporate information from different sources (multi-modality) and the unavailability of large datasets to train the models on. The main goal of this work was thus to make a contribution in this field by comparing deep learning with traditional machine learning techniques.

Due to the small dataset size, special methods, such as data augmentation and transfer learning were used when testing deep learning methods. Moreover, multi-modality and temporal evolution were considered by considering several fusion strategies, both at image level, feature level, and decision level.

Traditional learning was able to achieve 92.86% accuracy when using only two shape features extracted from the PTV. This comes, however, at the cost of not recommending surgery to a patient that should undergone this procedure. When using automatically extracted features, 100% accuracy was attained, perfectly classifying all of the examples. The architecture achieving this result was VGG-16, used to extract deep features from CT scans who are then classified with Classification ensembles. A paired-sample t-test applied to these two results, has proven that these results are not statistically significant.

This work represents some preliminary experiments and there are still some directions for the future. The first and most important is to validate the conclusion with bigger datasets. Next, it would be interesting to experiment with 3D deep learning strategies since here only 2D ones were used. If one decides that 2D methods are better, for being faster or more accurate, it would be interesting to develop a method to automatically select a slice from the volume (or a method to combine the results on several slices). For this, inspiration may be drawn from previous work on detection using deep learning or Bayesian surprise [6], [9]. Data fusion at input level for deep learning (for instance, inserting a different image type in each channel) will also be explored [7]. Data augmentation with anatomic considerations [7] and oversampling [8], [17] might help overcoming the data imbalance problem (64%

of the patients in the dataset had a complete pathological response, while 36% had an incomplete response). For being a medical application, we are also aware of the importance of interpretability [1].

In summary, we have explored various machine learning techniques in a biomedical context with the aim of advancing the state of the art in the field of computer vision in esophageal cancer. We do foresee, however, that the observation here made may be also applicable to other fields that also face the same difficulties, such as multi-modality and few labelled data.

REFERENCES

[1] José P. Amorim, Inês Domingues, Pedro H. Abreu, and João Santos. Interpreting Deep Learning Models for Ordinal Problems. *European Symposium on Artificial Neural Networks, Computational Intelligence and Machine Learning*, 1(1):25–27, 2018.

[2] A Amyar, S Ruan, I Gardin, C Chatelain, P Decazes, and R Modzelewski. 3-D RPET-NET: Development of a 3-D PET Imaging Convolutional Neural Network for Radiomics Analysis and Outcome Prediction. *IEEE Transactions on Radiation and Plasma Medical Sciences*, 3(2):225–231, mar 2019.

[3] Roelof J. Beukinga, Jan B. Hulshoff, Lisanne V. van Dijk, Christina T. Muijs, Johannes G.M. Burgerhof, Gursah Kats-Ugurlu, Riemer H.J.A. Slart, Cornelis H. Slump, Véronique E.M. Mul, and John Th.M. Plukker. Predicting Response to Neoadjuvant Chemoradiotherapy in Esophageal Cancer with Textural Features Derived from Pretreatment 18 F-FDG PET/CT Imaging. *Journal of Nuclear Medicine*, 58(5):723–729, may 2017.

[4] Freddie Bray, Jacques Ferlay, Isabelle Soerjomataram, Rebecca L Siegel, Lindsey A Torre, and Ahmedin Jemal. Global cancer statistics 2018: GLOBOCAN estimates of incidence and mortality worldwide for 36 cancers in 185 countries. *CA: A Cancer Journal for Clinicians*, 68(6):394–424, nov 2018.

[5] Jaime S Cardoso, Ricardo Sousa, and Ines Domingues. Ordinal Data Classification Using Kernel Discriminant Analysis: A Comparison of Three Approaches. In *11th International Conference on Machine Learning and Applications*, pages 473–477. IEEE, dec 2012.

[6] I Domingues and J S Cardoso. Mass detection on mammogram images: a first assessment of deep learning techniques. In *19th Portuguese Conference on Pattern Recognition*, page 2 pages, 2013.

[7] Ines Domingues, Pedro Henriques Abreu, and Joao Santos. Bi-Rads Classification of Breast Cancer: A New Pre-Processing Pipeline for Deep Models Training. In *2018 25th IEEE International Conference on Image Processing (ICIP)*, number Norte 2020, pages 1378–1382, oct 2018.

[8] Ines Domingues, Jose P. Amorim, Pedro Henriques Abreu, Hugo Duarte, and Joao Santos. Evaluation of Oversampling Data Balancing Techniques in the Context of Ordinal Classification. In *International Joint Conference on Neural Networks (IJCNN)*, number July, pages 1–8. IEEE, 2018.

[9] Ines Domingues and Jaime S. Cardoso. Using Bayesian surprise to detect calcifications in mammogram images. In *36th Annual International Conference of the IEEE Engineering in Medicine and Biology Society*, pages 1091–1094, aug 2014.

[10] Inês Domingues, Gisèle Pereira, Pedro Martins, Hugo Duarte, João Santos, and Pedro Henriques Abreu. Using deep learning techniques in medical imaging: a systematic review of applications on CT and PET. *Artificial Intelligence Review*, nov 2019.

[11] Ines Domingues, Ines Lucena Sampaio, Hugo Duarte, Joao A. M. Santos, and Pedro H. Abreu. Computer Vision in Esophageal Cancer: A Literature Review. *IEEE Access*, 7:103080–103094, 2019.

[12] J Ferlay, I Soerjomataram, and M Ervik. GLOBOCAN 2012v1.0, Cancer Incidence and Mortality Worldwide, 2013.

[13] Jorge Filipe Santos Ferreira, Inês Domingues, and João Santos. Classifying very small multi-modal data: application oesophagic early-stage cancers. *25th Portuguese Conference on Pattern Recognition (RECPAD)*, 2019.

[14] Kieran Foley, John Findlay, and Vicky Goh. Novel imaging techniques in staging oesophageal cancer. *Best Practice and Research in Clinical Gastroenterology*, 2018.

[15] Chunfeng Lian, Su Ruan, Thierry Denœux, Fabrice Jardin, and Pierre Vera. Selecting radiomic features from FDG-PET images for cancer treatment outcome prediction. *Medical Image Analysis*, 32:257–268, aug 2016.

[16] Chunfeng Lian, Su Ruan, Thierry Denoux, and Pierre Vera. Outcome prediction in tumour therapy based on Dempster-Shafer theory. In *IEEE 12th International Symposium on Biomedical Imaging (ISBI)*, pages 63–66, apr 2015.

[17] Francisco Marques, Hugo Duarte, João Santos, Inês Domingues, José P. Amorim, and Pedro H. Abreu. An iterative oversampling approach for ordinal classification. In *Proceedings of the 34th ACM/SIGAPP Symposium on Applied Computing*, pages 771–774, New York, NY, USA, apr 2019. ACM.

[18] Ana Catarina Oliveira, Inês Domingues, Hugo Duarte, João Santos, and Pedro H. Abreu. Going Back to Basics on Volumetric Segmentation of the Lungs in CT: A Fully Image Processing Based Technique. In *Iberian Conference on Pattern Recognition and Image Analysis (IbPRIA)*, pages 322–334. Springer, Cham, 2019.

[19] Martin C S Wong, Willie Hamilton, David C Whiteman, Johnny Y Jiang, Youlin Qiao, Franklin D H Fung, Harry H X Wang, Philip W Y Chiu, Enders K W Ng, Justin C Y Wu, Jun Yu, Francis K L Chan, and Joseph J Y Sung. Global Incidence and mortality of oesophageal cancer and their correlation with socioeconomic indicators temporal patterns and trends in 41 countries. *Scientific Reports*, 8(1):4522, dec 2018.

[20] Cheng-Kun Yang, Joe Chao-Yuan Yeh, Wei-Hsiang Yu, Ling-I. Chien, Ko-Han Lin, Wen-Sheng Huang, and Po-Kuei Hsu. Deep Convolutional Neural Network-Based Positron Emission Tomography Analysis Predicts Esophageal Cancer Outcome. *Journal of Clinical Medicine*, 8(6):844, jun 2019.

[21] Zhining Yang, Binghui He, Xinyu Zhuang, Xiaoying Gao, Dandan Wang, Mei Li, Zhixiong Lin, and Ren Luo. CT-based radiomic signatures for prediction of pathologic complete response in esophageal squamous cell carcinoma after neoadjuvant chemoradiotherapy. *Journal of Radiation Research*, 60(4):538–545, jul 2019.

[22] Hao Zhang, Shan Tan, Wengen Chen, Seth Kligerman, Grace Kim, Warren D. D'Souza, Mohan Suntharalingam, and Wei Lu. Modeling Pathologic Response of Esophageal Cancer to Chemoradiation Therapy Using Spatial-Temporal 18F-FDG PET Features, Clinical Parameters, and Demographics. *International Journal of Radiation Oncology*Biology*Physics*, 88(1):195–203, jan 2014.

9 783384 243188